The Principles and Practice of MOXIBUSTION

A fully illustrated guide to the theory and therapeutic techniques of moxibustion — the application of heat to acupuncture points.

The Principles and Practice of MOXIBUSTION

A Guide to the Therapeutic Application of Heat to Acupuncture Points

by

ROGER NEWMAN TURNER
B.Ac., N.D., D.O., M.B.Ac.A.

and

ROYSTON H. LOW
Ph.D., Dr.Ac., N.D., D.O., F.B.Ac.A.

Illustrations by Giles Newman Turner

THORSONS PUBLISHERS LIMITED
Wellingborough, Northamptonshire

First published in 1981

British Library Cataloguing in Publication Data

Low, Royston H.
The principles and practice of moxibustion
1. Acupuncture
I. Title II. Turner, R. Newman
615.8'92 RM184

ISBN 0-7225-0675-9

Typeset by Harper Phototypesetters, Northampton.
Printed and bound in Great Britain by
Biddles Limited, Guildford, Surrey.

CONTENTS

This book is dedicated to our wives and children,
Eunice, Ian and Christopher Low, and Birgid, Nicole
and Julian Newman Turner, whose patience and
endurance have made it possible.

ACKNOWLEDGEMENTS

The preparation of a textbook on a specialized topic, such as moxibustion, must, inevitably, draw upon knowledge and experience far beyond that of its authors. The debt we owe to the many acupuncturists whose wisdom and insight have been freely shared at conferences and informal gatherings in many parts of the world is considerable. We cannot name individually the many friends we have made in countries as diverse as China, Japan, Philippines, India, Sri Lanka, Australia, Kenya, Holland, France, U.S.A. and Canada, but we can acknowledge the contribution they have made to the field of acupuncture and moxibustion.

If particular parts of the world of acupuncture are to be singled out, we would like to express our special gratitude to our friends and colleagues in the Academy of Traditional Chinese Medicine, Peking, and to our fellow members of the British Acupuncture Association, who have been the vanguard in the establishment of acupuncture and moxibustion in this country. We have also received much help and encouragement from our colleagues in the British College of Acupuncture, and in particular the Dean Emeritus, Mr Keith Lamont (Dr.Ac.).

In this context we should also mention our special debt of gratitude to Dr J. Lavier who gave the first organized post-graduate instruction on acupuncture in this country, which led to the foundation of the Acupuncture Research Association and the B.A.A.

Undoubtedly the most difficult task in preparation of the manuscript is that of the typist who was required to cope with Chinese names and reproduce point numbers and tables with absolute accuracy. The typing of the various drafts was accomplished with aplomb by Mrs Angela Spencer, often working under the distracting conditions of a busy acupuncture clinic office, and these words cannot possibly express our gratitude to her.

Finally, we should like to thank Mr John Hardaker, Editorial Director of Thorsons Publishers Limited, who, in asking us to undertake this project, encouraged us to explore still further and discover even more of the value and potential of moxibustion than we had been aware of at the outset.

ROGER NEWMAN TURNER AND
ROYSTON H. LOW
London 1981

INTRODUCTION

The enthusiasm and euphoria that have accompanied the growth in the West of that branch of Oriental medicine known as acupuncture have tended to obscure some of the essential adjuncts to this great therapeutic system. The adoption of the term 'acupuncture' (Gr. *acu* = needle, *punctere* = pierce), or its European equivalents, has served to give greater emphasis to the use of the needles than the Chinese term of 'Chen-Chiu' (needle-moxa).

The two modalities are indivisible and, when human disease is considered from a traditional viewpoint—which seems the most comprehensive approach—no physician could be adequately equipped to deal with it without both at his disposal. Needle and moxibustion techniques are complementary.

What, then, is the justification for a textbook devoted primarily to moxibustion? Firstly, as cited above, there has been a pre-occupation with the use of needles to the exclusion of moxibustion. Moxa is regarded by some practitioners as being old-fashioned and messy—it does not suit the clean, sterile image of modern medicine. Patients, particularly those with chronic disorders and diseases of cold and damp environments, have been the victims of this attitude. Foremost among the advantages of moxibustion are its capacity to counteract the influence of cold or damp conditions on the body and its reinforcing properties in states of depletion or weakness. It also has the advantage over needles of not transmitting infection.

The indisputable value of moxibustion in the management of chronic disorders, conditions of deficiency, and those aggravated by adverse climatic conditions, can be well corroborated by those practitioners who include it in their armamentarium. The prevalence of disease due to inadequate cellular nutrition is so much more pronounced in modern society. Reinforcement techniques, whether nutritional (herbs, supplements), or energetic, are so often required and moxa is a tool of great efficacy in achieving this. The drying and warming properties of moxa complement the sedative, or 'moving', effects of needling procedures. The latter 'move' energy within the system whereas moxa supplies energy from an external source.

This interpretation of the comparison between needles and moxa is based on the Tsang-Fu (Yin/Yang) concepts, an understanding of which is essential to the effective use of moxibustion, but even on a more materialistic basis, the use of heat as a method of pain regulation is a well established procedure. The physiological responses to moxibustion are preparatory to a general elevation of body immunity.

The use of heat as a therapeutic modality is clouded in the mists of antiquity. Cauterization was probably used systematically long before the discovery of needles and the more precise location of the acupuncture points. Its development was in parallel with needling as a complementary system with regional emphasis dictated by climatic variations. In China, the higher and colder parts of the continent saw greater use of moxibustion and more variety in the ways of applying heat to the body. In spite of the development of more sophisticated electrical devices, the traditional use of dried Artemisia still remains the most popular and economical way of applying moxibustion. Its unique properties have yet to be fully explained.

This book aims to provide a comprehensive guide to the various methods and techniques of moxibustion, as well as presenting the practitioner with an outline of its chief therapeutic applications. It seeks to place the use of moxa in its proper perspective and it must be emphasized that, whilst dealing exclusively with moxibustion, the authors do not advocate this as a comprehensive therapeutic system. In order to use the recommendations and formulae in this book it is essential to have a full understanding of acupuncture theory and practice, to be familiar with its diagnostic principles and with the indications for selection of needles and/or moxa in treatment.

With these essential foundations, however, it is to be hoped that this textbook will provide a definitive reference work for every practitioner dedicated to furthering the development of a health care system that is compatible with the subtle and intricate processes of the human body.

1

HISTORY AND DEVELOPMENT OF MOXIBUSTION

The therapeutic properties of heat have probably been known to man since his most primitive beginnings. The comfort derived from the warmth of the sun would have been evident before the discovery of fire and the attribution to it of ritualistic significance. But the difference between symbolism and practical benefit must soon have become clear for, according to Wang Xuetai:

> In primitive society, when people were warming themselves by fire, they accidentally discovered that by applying heat to the abdominal area they could relieve symptoms of abdominal pain, distension, and fullness.[1]

Thus moxibustion, the application of heat to a specific area of the body for the purpose of treating illness, was evolved. It later became an integral part of the Chinese system of medicine, incorporating the use of needles, herbs, hydrotherapy, and dietetics.

Although much of the philosophy and practical knowledge which underlies these methods of treatment evolved in China, the term 'moxibustion' is derived from the Japanese, *Moe kusa*, meaning 'burning herb'.[2]

The development of acupuncture and moxibustion later became integrated. In China there is evidence of cauterization being used in parallel with needling techniques using sharp stones (Bian stones), some 10,000 years ago.[3] Various materials were used to apply the heat, ranging from dry leaves and twigs to charcoal, chopsticks, and sulphur, but, eventually, the dried leaves of *Artemisia vulgaris* became the most popular.

Artemisia vulgaris (Mugwort, Chinese Wormwood) is widely distributed throughout the Far East and much of Europe (see figure 1). The sun-dried leaves were generally powdered to a fine tobacco consistency and applied to the acupuncture points and other areas of the body, then ignited and allowed to burn until they became too hot. The heat and consistency of the herb were found to be more suitable than other forms of cauterization. Various other herbs were, however, incorporated for their therapeutic properties.

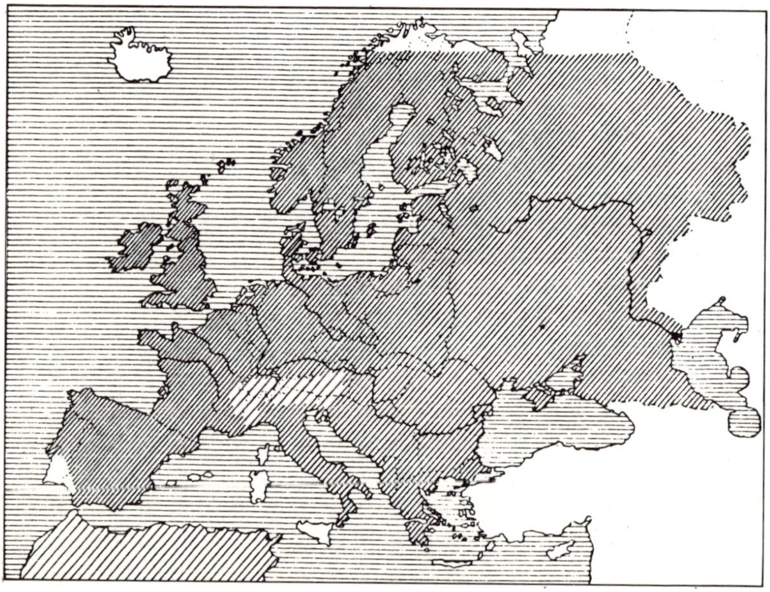

Figure 1. European distribution of *Artemisia vulgaris, L.* (from *Lehrbuch der Biologischen Heilmittel* by G. Madaus).

Indirect methods of heating, using garlic and ginger slices, were discovered, and sticks of moxa, called 'Magic Sticks of Thunder and Fire', were also used. There are now many different ways of applying moxibustion and these will be considered more fully in Chapter 2.

Ancient Texts

The earliest use of moxa sticks is recorded in a book called *Magic Remedy*, published at a time when the mystical properties of the treatment were thought most significant. Moxibustion had its obvious, more practical use, however, for it is recorded that 'burning dried moxa leaves against mosquitoes, or throwing ground moxa leaves into a cesspool or latrine, as insecticide, has been a common practice from ancient time'. As early as the third century A.D. books on moxibustion appeared bearing titles such as *Chao's Moxibustion Method*, and *Moxibustion for Consumptive Diseases*, and *New Book on Surgical Moxibustion*.[5]

Some early physicians attempted to develop moxibustion as an independent system because of its simplicity but, as Wang Xuetai points out, it is indivisible from the total system of Chinese medicine.[6] Nevertheless, such was the degree of specialization in the art that in 1128 Chuang Cho published a treatise entitled *Kao Huang Chiu Fa* [On Moxibustion at Kao Huang (Bl.38) Point].[7]

Chinese medicine went through various stages of development as the social system changed from slavery to feudalism which, in turn, began to crumble in the time of the Warring States (475-221 B.C.). It was during this period that the *Huang Di Nei Jing* was published. This Canon of Internal Medicine was a distillation of the knowledge accumulated up to that time, set in the form of a discussion between the Yellow Emperor, Huang Di, and his physician, Chi Po. It is one of the few medical texts of the time to have survived and it established the foundation for the basic theories of Chinese medicine, including moxibustion, which have been applied to this day.

The *Nei Jing* consists of two parts, the *Sou Wen* (Plain Questions) and the *Ling Shu* (Canon of Acupuncture). In the *Sou Wen*, under the chapter 'Treatise on Suitable Prescriptions with Different Methods' we find the following passage:

> . . . moxibustion originated from the north, as the northern places are shut off from heaven and earth, and where high and mountainous areas are attacked by piercing cold wind and are surrounded by much ice. People there live in camps in the wilderness and subsist on milk. They become ill when invaded by the cold, and moxibustion is the method of treatment.

That last statement summarizes the essential diagnostic and

therapeutic indications for moxibustion — the prevention and dispersal of diseases due to cold and damp. It also suggests more strongly the regional emphasis on the different aspects of Chinese medicine — the greater use of warming and supplying procedures, with moxibustion and herbs, in the colder regions, and of dispersing and draining techniques (needles and cupping) in the lower-lying plains and coastal areas. The monks of the mountainous areas are said to have fortified themselves for long journeys by the application of moxa to Tsusanli, St 36.

The *Nei Jing* was a compilation of knowledge by various authorities at the time, but another text held in high regard is the *Shang-han Tsa-ping Lun* (Treatise in Sixteen Chapters on Various Ailments Caused by the Cold) attributed to Chang Chung Ching (born circa 160 A.D.), who is regarded as the Chinese Hippocrates.[8] Chang Chung Ching also gave the first clear differentiation between Yin and Yang.

Establishment of Principles

The firm establishment of moxibustion as a universal method of treatment led to various explanations of its effect, and some dogmas over its application were passed from generation to generation without much question as to their validity.

Some rules, such as those concerning the optimum number of moxas and forbidden points, are still given credence by many practitioners, although it is often difficult to give a satisfactory rationale for adherence to such beliefs. Many of the forbidden points may well have been established for cosmetic and fashion reasons (see *Appendix 1*). In the ancient times direct moxibustion was more commonly used and the blisters resulting from this might have been aggravated by the friction of tight clothing over certain points.

Whilst the new wave of experimental work resulted in the disproving of some absolute rules, and the debunking of some 'forbidden points', it is more difficult to be definitive about other observations of the ancients, such as the treatise of the Warring States period which says, 'In treating a disease seven years old, use three year old moxa.' The use of seasoned moxa in stubborn cases seems to have been common practice and may be physiologically more suitable when considered on a Tsang-Fu basis.

The efficacy and the survival of older methods in the face of modern technology, bears witness to the existence of as yet unexplained therapeutic properties in the many different forms of moxibustion now in common use.

SUMMARY OF ADVANTAGES AND DISADVANTAGES OF MOXIBUSTION

Advantages	*Disadvantages*
Warming; ideal for cold, damp conditions. Aseptic. Ease of administration. Patient can be treated in any position. Fainting risk minimal. Suitable for patients who are: afraid of needles, chronically sick, children.	Risk of burns with frail, sensitive, diabetic, and hemiplegic patients. Untidy. Time consuming.

REFERENCES

[1]Wang Xuetai. 'A Research on the Origin and Development of Chinese Acupuncture and Moxibustion.' National Symposia of Acupuncture and Moxibustion and Acupuncture Anaesthesia. Beijing, June 1979.

[2]Heuser, G. D., and Pennell, R. J., *The How To Seminar of Acupuncture For Physicians*. (Independence, Missouri, 1973).

[3]Wang Xuetai, *op. cit.*

[4]Fu Wei-kang. *The Story of Chinese Acupuncture and Moxibustion* (Foreign Languages Press, Peking 1975).

[5]Wang Xuetai, *op. cit.*

[6]Wang Xuetai. Personal communication (July 1980).

[7]Gwei-Djen, L., and Needham, J., *Celestial Lancets*, (Cambridge University Press, 1980).

[8]Huard, P., and Wong, M., *Chinese Medicine*, (Weidenfeld and Nicolson, London 1968).

2

METHODS OF MOXIBUSTION

The application of heat is probably the oldest form of treatment devised by man and, in spite of very little fundamental change in its method of administration, it still remains one of the most effective. From the earliest times various ways of applying heat were used, ranging from hot stones and sticks to canisters containing hot water or combustible material, but it was soon discovered that the most suitable substance for the purpose of moxibustion was the dried herb Artemisia.

Artemisia

Artemisia is a perennial herb of the family Compositae (Daisy family). The most common variety found in Europe is *A. vulgaris* (Mugwort, Wormwood) which reaches a height of four to five feet and grows on waste ground and roadsides.[1] Other varieties of Mugwort are also found and cultivated in China and Japan where commercial production of moxa is carried out.

Chinese Mugwort (*A. veriotorum*) is more aromatic. *A. abrotanum* and *A. capillaris* are also used.[2] In Chinese the plant is called *Ai* and the powder prepared from it is known as *Airong*.

The constituents of Artemisia are a volatile oil, resin, tannin and artemisin (a bitter principle).[3] Medicinally it is valued as a nervine, tonic, febrifuge, anti-epileptic and emmenagogue.[2, 3]

Preparation of Moxa

Traditionally Artemisia was picked in the fifth lunar month and dried for three years. Sun-dried moxa was regarded as being more efficacious, possibly because of the powers attributed to sunlight from early times.

The mid-ribs are stripped out of the leaves and they are then ground in a mortar and pestle to form moxa punk, or tinder, of a fine tobacco or wool-like consistency.

In China other drugs or plants are mixed with the Artemisia such as *Aquilaria agallocha*, *Rosa banksiae*, *Pistacia lentiscus*, dried ginger, and ant-eater.

One of the authors harvests his own Artemisia in June or July when the flowers are just ripe, and uses both leaves and flower buds which are placed in a coffee grinder for about twenty seconds. The dust is then sifted out and the remaining moss, or wool, is used.[3]

Moxa Wool or Punk

The resultant wool, or moxa punk, is of a dry fibrous consistency with self-adherent properties which make it suitable for separating into loosely packed pinches of various sizes. Moxa burns at an even rate without flame which makes it a suitable way of administering heat gently.

There are two principal methods of moxibustion, direct and indirect, and moxa punk is prepared and applied in various ways appropriate to each method. For direct moxibustion, a finer grade of punk is preferred, whilst for indirect moxibustion the coarser type, which tends to have more ribs and stalks in the mixture, is adequate. The most easily obtainable Chinese moxa punk tends to be coarse, whilst the finer grade is prepared in Japan.

Moxa punk is applied to the points directly in small cones moulded by the fingers to the size of a rice grain, date stone, or thumb nail or broad bean (see Figure 2). The amount of wool, and therefore the time for which it burns, is known as a 'zhuan'. The top of the cone is ignited with a flame, or incense stick and the cone allowed to burn down until it becomes too hot. In some forms of direct moxibustion the cone is allowed to burn the skin and form a blister, the technique being known as *Aizhu jiufa*.

Moxa punk is also used for indirect methods of cauterization on garlic, or ginger slices, salt, or medicinal cake (see page 29).

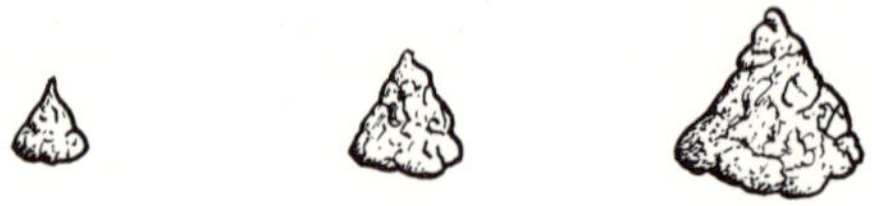

(a) (b) (c)

Figure 2. Moxa cones of various sizes—(a) rice grain size; (b) date stone size; and (c) broad bean size.

Moxa Rolls

These were developed as a more convenient method of indirect cauterization in the Ming and Ching dynasties when they were known as 'Magic Sticks of Thunder and Fire', or 'Tai Yi Magic Sticks'.

Moxa rolls (*Ai juan jiu*) are prepared by mixing moxa punk with other ingredients and then rolling them tightly, with paper, into a cigar-shaped stick of approximately 20cm (8½ ins) by 1-2cm (¾ ins) in diameter—20cm = 6 cun, and each cun burns for ten or twelve minutes (see *Glossary*). The thin inner wrapping is of a mulberry skin paper secured with egg white and the outer layer, of thicker paper, is applied and sealed with adhesive.

Some more elaborate traditional recipes are used for specialized applications, two of which are given below.

1. *Lightening Cauterization* (*Leihuo jiufa*). A mixture of 8.5g (⅓ oz) each of *Aquillaria agallocha*, *Rosa banksiae*, *Pistacia lentiscus*, *Artemisia capillaris*, *Zingiberis* (Ginger) and *Squama manitis* (ant-eater) with a little musk and 50g (2 oz) of moxa powder is prepared. This is rolled tightly in one thin and one thick sheet of paper and sealed with egg white. Application: a coarse cloth about 30cms (12 ins) square is folded seven or eight times and placed over the point. The ignited end of the roll is placed against it and heat penetrates through the holes in the cloth.

2. *Tai Yi Spiritual Moxibustion* (*Taiyishen jiufa*). This is used as above, but the roll is made of the following ingredients: moxa powder 8.5g (⅓ oz), sulphur 5.5g (⅕ oz), musk, *Pistacia lentiscus*, myrrh, *Jambosa caryophyllus*, *Santalum album*,

Cinnamomum cassia (branch), *Angelica anomala*, *Eucommia ulmoides*, Orange peel, *Gleditsohia horrida*, *Angelica grosserrata*, *Asarum sieboldi*, and ant-eater. Some authorities add 3g ($^1/_{10}$ oz) *Conioselinun unvittam* and a whole dried scorpion is added to the mixture.[5]

The most widely used moxa rolls are those available commercially from China and Japan. Tai Yi and Nien Ying are stronger and faster burning combinations of moxa wool and other herbal ingredients. Mild moxibustion rolls have a slower combustion rate and less intensity of heat which makes them suitable for patients with more delicate constitutions, such as children, or the elderly.

Japanese Moxa Rolls

Refillable Moxa Device. In addition to various paper-bound moxa rolls, the Japanese have devised refillable moxa rolls con-

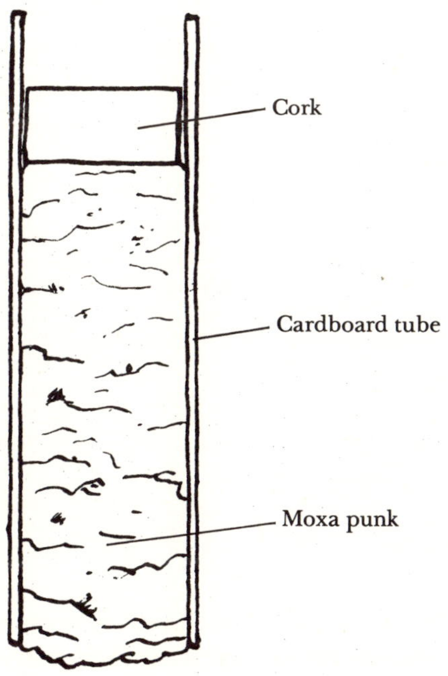

Figure 3. Refillable moxa tube from Japan.

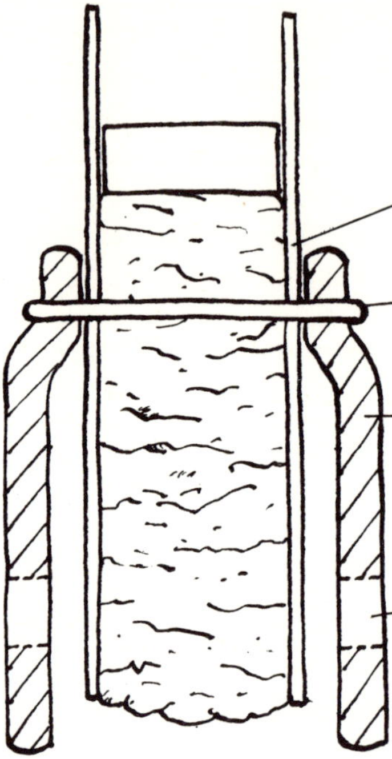

Figure 4. Moxa roll with hood.

sisting of a stout cardboard tube which is packed with moxa punk (see Figure 3). A cork in one end enables the moxa to be pushed through the tube exposing sufficient to be ignited at the burning end. This is a more economical method of moxibustion.

The refillable moxa tube can be used in conjunction with a moxa hood (see Figure 4). This consists of a wooden cover with hand grip at one end designed to hold moxa rolls. The roll is ignited and placed in the hood with the burning surface adjusted to a suitable height.

The advantage of the moxa device with hood is that application can be more carefully regulated. With the base of the hood resting on the skin there is greater stability and the distance between the roll and the skin surface can be consistently set. The hood also prevents the smoke getting in the practitioner's face!

Hood devices are also manufactured with handles to enable self-application to areas such as the back and shoulders.

Akabane Sticks (Greensticks). This is a type of incense stick prepared from a finely ground combination of herbs and mineral ingredients. A paste is formed into sticks of approximately 3mm ($^1/_8$ in) in diameter. They are available as finer sticks (usually green) or a more sturdy type (brown).

Akabane sticks are so named because of their use in the Akabane Test (see *Appendix 3*). They have the advantage of applying a more localized heat for points in anatomically restricted areas such as the natal cleft (e.g., Chang Chiang, Gv 1, or Huiyin, VC 1), or on the extremities (e.g., Tsing points). They are also suitable for the 'pecking' technique where a large number of very local moxas are called for. A typical example would be the use of a special point above the ulnar styloid in the treatment of hemiplegia which calls for a minimum of fifty moxas.

Akabane, or greensticks, are also most suitable for igniting moxa cones.

Adhesive Cones. A form of indirect moxibustion is given by means of various types of small cardboard tube containing sufficient moxa wool for one application. One end of the tube is adhesive so that the device can be fixed over the point and ignited (see Figure 5). These are suitable for self-administration.

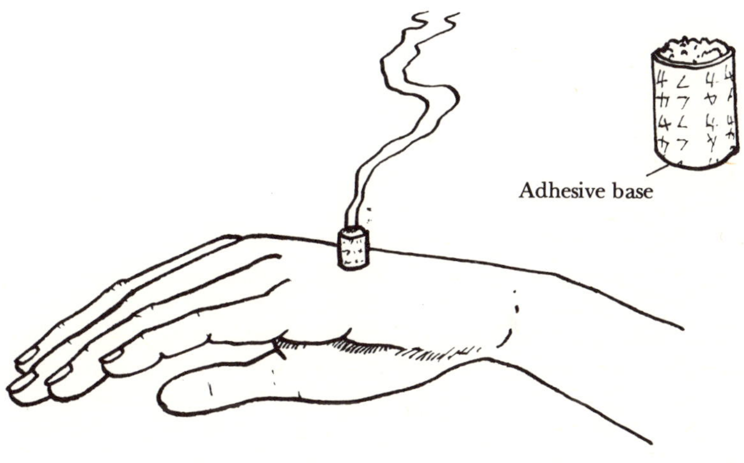

Figure 5. Adhesive tubes for indirect moxibustion.

Moxa Frames

For a more generalized application of heat a device widely used in Chinese hospitals consists of a square wooden frame about 15cm (6 ins) across and 7.5cm (3 ins) deep, with a base of fine wire mesh about 2.5cm (1 in) up to resemble a fine sieve (see Figure 6).

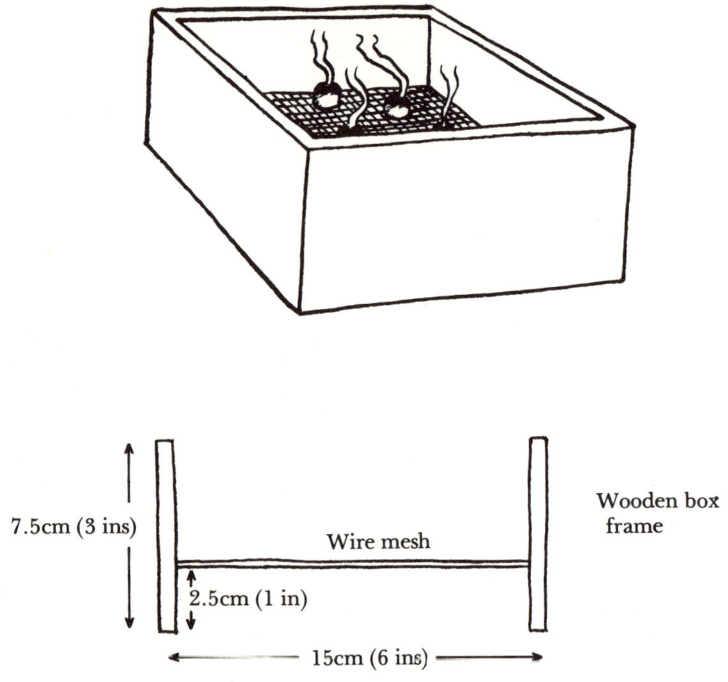

Figure 6. Wooden frames for moxibustion to large areas.

Several large pieces of moxa roll are placed in it and ignited, a lid is placed on top, to keep the heat in, and the device is placed on the abdomen or other larger areas requiring treatment. It is used particularly in the treatment of gastro-intestinal conditions.

Warm Canister Moxibustion

Special metal containers which can be filled with moxa wool and medicinal powders. They are flat or conical in shape and are moved gently over the points or the area to be treated.

Other Types of Cauterization

Warming devices are available which consist of a small electrical element capable of generating a radiant heat. They have the advantage of cleanliness but the disadvantage of needing a power source. The warming properties cannot resemble those of the herbal combination of the moxa rolls.

Other types of cauterization are referred to by some authorities. Chung and Lee[5] refer to 'blistering therapy' using herbs and spices. We shall, however, confine ourselves to moxibustion in the context of warming with the dried herb and allied preparations.

REFERENCES

[1]Fitter, R. and Fitter, A., *The Wild Flowers of Britain and Northern Europe* (Collins, London 1974).

[2]Madaus, G., *Lehrbuch der Biologischen Heilmittel, I*, page 601 (George Olms Verlag, Hildesheim, 1976).

[3]Steinmetz, E. F., *Codex Vegetabilis* (Amsterdam, 1957).

[4]Low, R. H., 'Prepare Your Own Moxa', British Acupuncture Association Conference, London, 1980.

[5]Heroldova, D., *Acupuncture and Moxibustion* (Czeckoslovak Academy of Sciences, Prague, 1968).

[6]Lee, J. F. and Cheung, C. S., *Current Acupuncture Therapy*, (Medical Book Publications, Hong Kong, 1978).

3

TECHNIQUES OF MOXIBUSTION

Having made a diagnostic assessment according to the Eight Principles and analysis of Yin-Yang equilibrium (see Chapter 5) the practitioner, if he has decided upon treatment with moxa, or combined techniques, such as heated needles, will need to select an appropriate method of moxibustion. This will depend upon the constitution of the patient and the location of the points selected for treatment. According to Yi Zhon Ji Jian:

> For treatment of various diseases by moxibustion, the fire must be necessarily sufficient and the Chi attained. Only then may cure be accomplished.[1]

There are two fundamental types of cauterization: that leaving blisters or marks (*Yu banhen jiu*) which is always direct, and that not leaving marks (*Wu banhen jiu*) which can be direct or indirect. It is, therefore, most convenient to classify moxibustion techniques according to whether they are direct or indirect.

Direct Moxibustion

This method (*Aizhu jiufa*) involves the use of moxa cones applied directly to the skin surface. The marking and non-marking methods are used.

Preparing the Cone

Roll a small amount of moxa punk between the fingers and compress it into a tight cone with a broad base. Traditionally the three sizes of moxa cone recommended were, rice grain (small), date stone (medium), and thumb nail or broad bean (large). The amount of moxa punk in the cone is known as a 'zhuan' which is, therefore, a measure of the time taken for a cone to burn.

Small cones generate little heat and are suitable for children and those of weaker constitution. They are also indicated where a precise but limited stimulus is required over more delicate areas. Larger cones generate a greater heat by burning for longer and may be used where the constitution is sturdy and a stronger stimulus is required. The more tightly compressed the moxa wool is, the greater the heat developed and the depth of penetration.

Position of Patient

The patient should be placed in a comfortable position either sitting or, preferably, lying. The likelihood of syncope while undergoing moxibustion is negligible, compared to the use of needles, but the possibility of a sudden vascular shunt, or movement of energy, in a patient of sensitive constitution must always be considered.

The points to be treated must be accessible to the practitioner and the patient placed in such a way as to permit the moxa cones to be placed securely on them. Ensure that there is no danger of the ignited cone falling onto delicate areas such as the eye.

Igniting the Cone

The cone is placed firmly on the point, which may be slightly moistened, if necessary, for adhesion. The tip of the cone should be ignited with a glowing taper, or green moxa stick. It is then allowed to burn down towards the skin. The duration of burning depends on whether the marking or non-marking method is used.

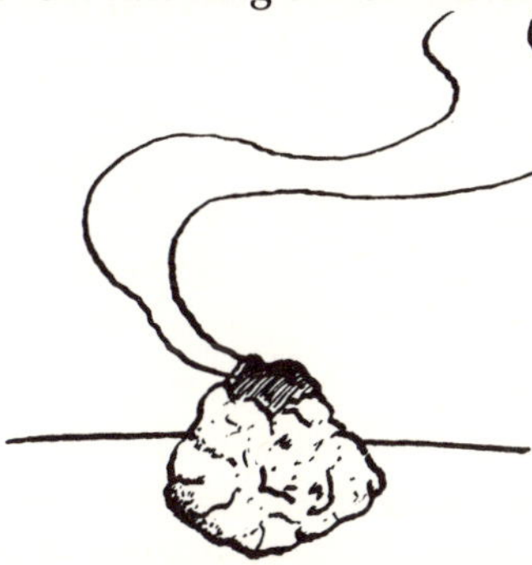

Figure 7. Direct moxibustion with cone.

If the *marking technique* is used, the cone is allowed to burn almost to the skin surface which will exhibit immediate erythema, or a wheal. The burned moxa ash is then removed into a receptacle. When a wheal, or blister, has appeared, which may require the application of several cones (6-8 zhuans), the area should be cleansed with cool boiled water and covered with a suitable ointment such as *Calendula officinalis*. If suppuration occurs the wound should be cleansed daily with a 10 per cent solution of Calendula tincture and the ointment applied to the margins until healing has taken place.

The counter-irritant effect of the blistering technique is stronger if suppuration occurs and may be increased by the application of extract of *Allium sativum* (Common Garlic). The patient should be advised of the possibility of suppuration and reassured as to its benefits. He should receive instructions in proper care of the wound to encourage scar-free healing.

Blistering moxibustion is not suitable for dark-skinned people as it may result in permanent depigmentation.

In the more usual practice of *non-marking* moxibustion the patient must advise the practitioner when the burning moxa cone is no longer tolerable. The initial sensation of gentle warmth will change to a sharper hot sensation which is when the cone should be removed. Repeat the process at each point, remembering that with each subsequent cone the threshold will be reached more rapidly. A diffuse erythema will remain, but gradually fades.

Duration and Number of Applications

Whilst older texts and many modern authorities make specific recommendations as to the number of zhuans to be used at each point, these serve only as approximate guidelines and moxibustion should always be adapted to the sensitivity and tolerance of the patient. It is more usual nowadays to moxa the point until a palpably distinct heat is retained by the skin for several minutes. There are certain conditions and formulas in which a specific number of zhuans must be applied. Some ancient texts recommended that the following guidelines be used.

> For thickly muscled areas such as shoulders, lower back, and buttocks, more applications are used; abdomen, arms and legs, slightly less; chest, head, face and fleshless parts of the extremities, few applications; for the old and young apply less; for those of weak constitution smaller cones must be applied for a longer time.[2]

Indirect Moxibustion

Moxibustion in which the punk does not have direct contact with the skin is done either with cones or with moxa rolls.

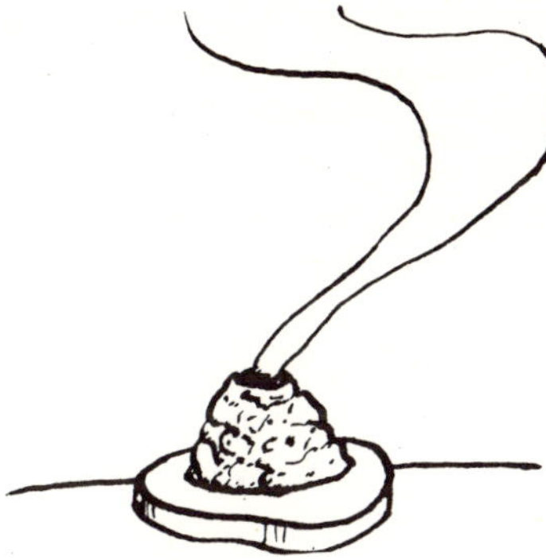

Figure 8. Indirect moxibustion with cone on garlic or ginger slice.

Indirect Moxa with Cones

The moxa cone is ignited on a layer of sliced herb or medicinal cake placed over the point (see Figure 8). The stimulus varies according to the substance used.

1. *On Ginger* (*Gejiang jiufa*). Slice of ginger 1-3 fen (see *Glossary*) thick, with tiny holes pierced in it, placed under cone. If the pain is too violent, remove until it subsides, then replace the cone and ginger and keep it there until the patient perspires and the point becomes red. There is danger of blistering if the heat is not regulated.
2. *On Garlic* (*Gesuan jiufa*). Used as above, but when the pain is felt it should not be removed. Used for chronic paralysis, or for the early stage of a carbuncle. In this latter condition, a piece of wet paper is put on the carbuncle, and on the spot where it dries out from the underlying inflammation one places a slice of garlic about 3 fen thick with the moxa cone on top. Change the garlic after 5 cones. If the carbuncle is painful, cauterize until the pain disappears: if not painful, cauterize until it becomes so. If no suppuration occurs, one can apply long-lasting cauterization. If the carbuncle has several heads, spread squashed garlic over it before applying the cone.

3. *On Bean-Cake* (*Gehing jiufa*). A cake is prepared of crushed bean, pepper, ginger, salt, and onion, 3 fen thick, and placed under the cone. If patient feels too hot, it may be removed for a while and then replaced. Keep it on until patient feels 'hot inside' and skin becomes red. Do not use in cases of suppuration.
4. *On Monk's Hood* (*Fuzi jiufa*). Monk's Hood is ground into a powder and mixed with a powder of *Bletilla hyacintha* and water to form a cake 3 fen thick. Place on sore area with moxa on top. When cake dries out, replace with another, until patient feels hot inside.
5. *On Salt* (*Geyan jiufa*). The navel is filled to the brim with fine salt on which the cone is placed. Garlic or ginger slice may also be placed on the salt. This method is used only on the navel, and was described mainly by Chi Shouyan and Cheng Danan. It is efficacious in cases of abdominal pain, and diarrhoea.
6. *On Clay* (*Huangtu jiufa*). Described by the authors above. Moxa is put on a cake of clay. It is used for eczema and skin diseases caused by humidity. Cauterize until the patient 'feels hot inside'.
7. *Aconite Cake*. Ground slices of Aconite root are mixed into a paste with yellow wine. A layer is placed over the point and the moxa cone is ignited on top of it.

Most of these methods of indirect moxibustion have a reinforcing effect to the basic heat stimulus of the moxa. They are used for symptom complexes of 'insufficient Yang'. Where the therapeutic power of the herb, such as ginger or garlic, is required with a milder stimulus, the effect may be tempered by placing the slice and moxa cone on several layers of gauze.

Moxa Rolls

Moxa rolls are more convenient than cones to use in reinforcing techniques. The patient may be treated in any position which is comfortable and it is possible to treat points on which it would be difficult to place a cone, including those which are covered by hair.

Moxa Roll Technique

Having selected a suitable roll, according to the constitution of the patient, the end is ignited to give an even red glow. It will generally be necessary to retract the outer paper so that the mixture in the tissue paper will glow with sufficient intensity to produce smoke. During administration of treatment the end of the roll should regularly be tapped into a receptacle to remove surplus ash.

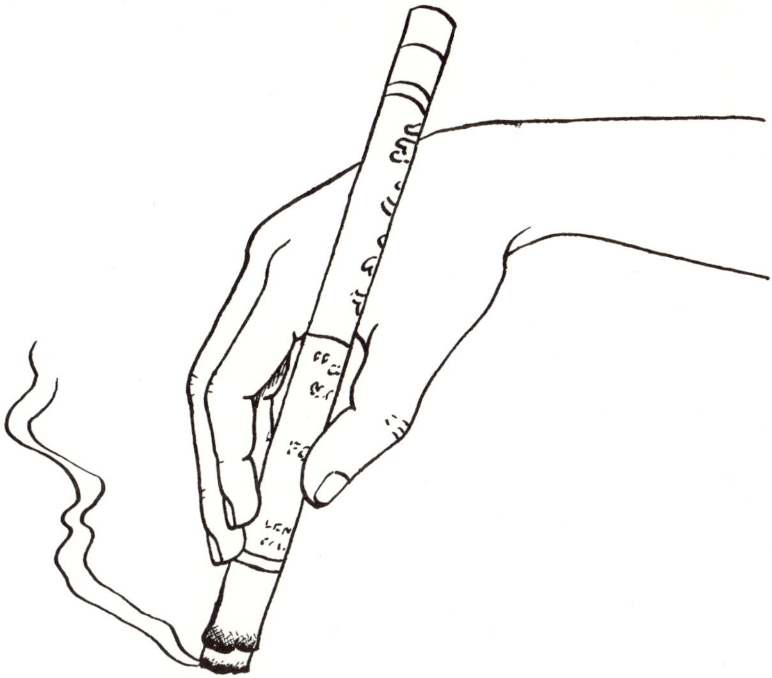

Figure 9. Holding the fuming moxa roll.

There are three methods of application:

1. *Warm cauterization* (*Wenhe jiufa*). The burning end is brought slowly nearer to the skin over the point — usually about ½-1 cun. It is allowed to fume for five to ten minutes. The patient feels a pleasant warmth but should advise the operator if the heat becomes intolerable. The technique is suitable for sedation. It is best applied with mild moxa rolls or the Japanese hood type of roll.

2. *Spreading or rotation method.* The ignited roll is brought to within ½-1 cun of the skin and then moved slowly to and fro across the affected area (see Figure 10). This is suitable for chronic disorders where a general reinforcement is required over an area which is suffering from the penetration of cold or damp perverse influences, such as the anterior aspect of the knee, covering the *Hsiyen* points, across the *Ba feng* points in arthritic disorders of the metatarso-phalangeal joints or, in cases of bronchitis and respiratory problems, in a line from Bl 37 to Bl 13, Gv 12, Bl 13, Bl 37 and back again.

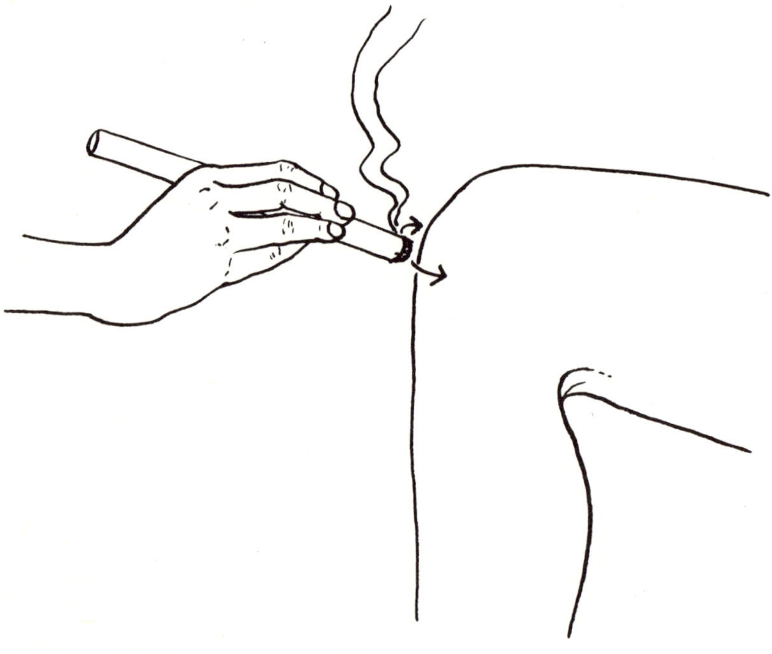

Figure 10. Spreading technique with moxa roll to Hsiyen points of knee.

Rotation technique is applied with a circular motion of the roll (see Figure 11). This is generally applied around a point which might be too sensitive for the direct or the sustained application of heat.

3. *Sparrow-peck cauterization* (*Quezhuo jiufa*). The lighted end of the roll is brought slowly near to and away from the skin so that the patient feels a pleasant warmth. It is used mostly for tonification and takes a shorter time than warm cauterization, usually 2-5 minutes.

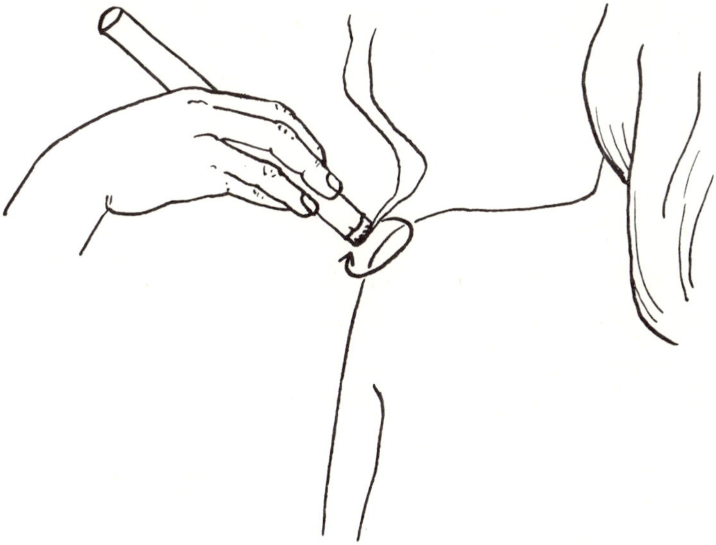

Figure 11. Rotation technique with moxa roll to Co15.

General Considerations in Moxa Roll Technique

For tonification of individual points with moxa rolls the most suitable technique is similar to the Sparrow-peck method. The moxa roll should be held ½-1 cun from the surface. If the roll is held in a pen grip the ulnar surface of the practitioner's hand should rest on the patient's skin for stability (see Figure 12). This is important in order to minimize the possibility of accidentally touching the patient's skin, particularly when the point becomes too hot and sudden movements are likely to occur.

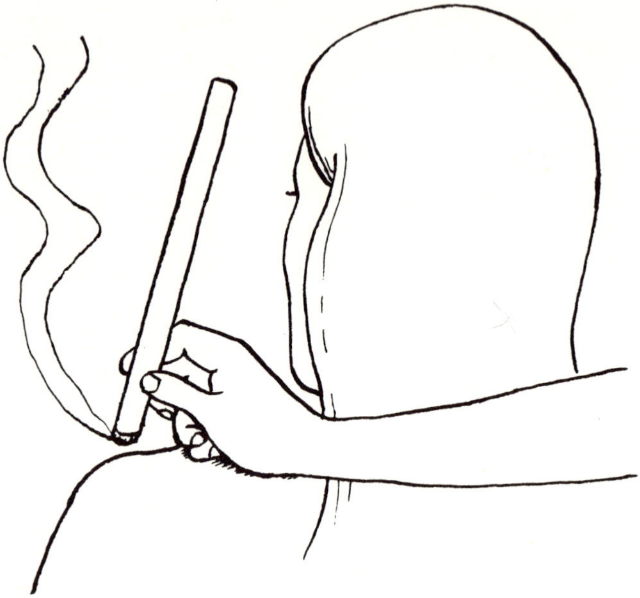

Figure 12. Applying the moxa roll. Note that the practitioner's hand is resting on the patient's skin for stability.

The patient should be instructed to state when the point becomes too hot, normally felt as a sudden sharp heat penetrating the skin. In order to avoid misunderstanding of other words during conversation it is preferable for the patient to indicate tolerance limit by simply saying 'hot'.

The moxa is withdrawn for three or four seconds and applied again as often as is necessary to attain the level of palpable heat retention. It will normally take three to ten seconds for a properly fuming roll to achieve tolerance limit at the first application and this will reduce to one or two seconds as the heat accumulates at the point.

Moxibustion to Hair-covered Points

With the indirect technique, using the moxa rolls, it is possible to apply moxibustion to points which are covered with hair. The point should be located and the hair parted as much as possible with the fingers. It is then held flat against the skin with the parted fingers and the fuming tip of the moxa roll is approximated to the point in the usual manner (see Figure 13).

This method prevents the hair being singed and is suitable for points such as *Paihui*, Gv 20, or, in hirsute individuals, *Shanchung*, Vc 17.

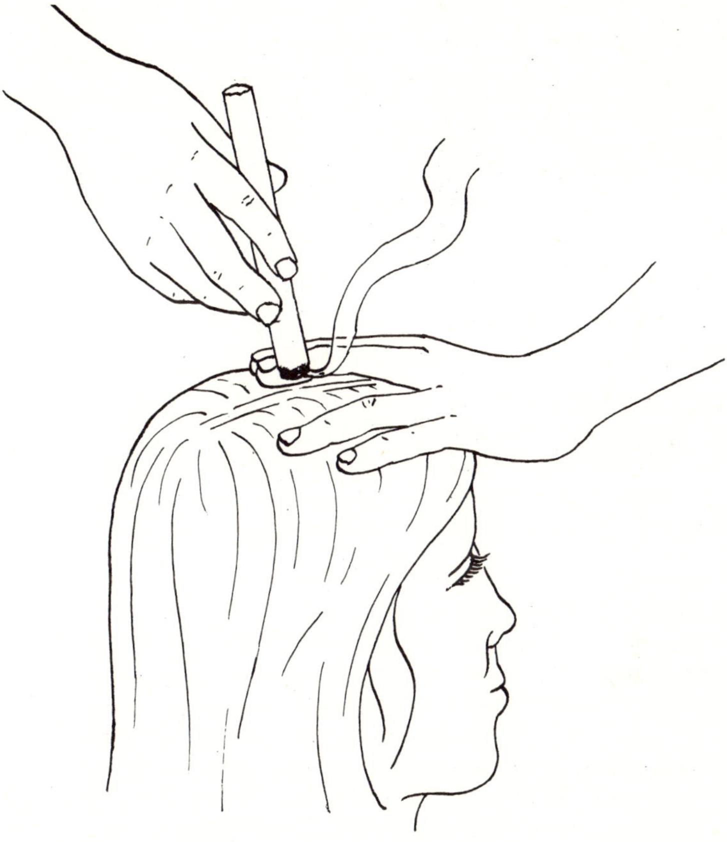

Figure 13. Moxibustion to points lying under hair.

Moxibustion for Paralysed Patients

Certain precautions must be taken when applying moxibustion to cases of hemiplegia. In spastic paralysis there will usually be a delayed but exaggerated motor response to the moxa stimulus.

If sensory response is diminished, the practitioner should place a finger close to the point being heated and endeavour to assess the tolerance limit by his own response to the heat.

Further Precautions in Moxa Roll Application

1. When treating abdominal points, remember that the muscles will tend to move towards the roll as the patient reacts to the heat. By resting on the abdomen the knuckles of your hand holding the moxa stick, you will feel the muscular contraction and avoid burning the patient's skin.
2. Do not allow ash to accumulate on the end of the stick as this may fall off on the skin of the patient and will also reduce the radiant heat.
3. Never move the moxa stick about over the eyes of the patient.
4. Exercise caution regarding clothing (especially nylon underwear), paper dressing towels, and blankets.
5. Always have an ash tray or non-flammable receptacle at hand.
6. Moxa rolls may be snuffed and stored in a candlestick holder, metal film cassette-holder or stainless steel moxa roll holder. Japanese moxa hood devices have an aluminum cap which fits over the end of the tube.

Heated Needle Techniques

A more precise stimulation is obtained by the use of heated needles. The needle is said to direct the warmth into the meridian and, in conditions due to devitalization of the Yong and Wei energy, such as chronic spinal problems, the technique is particularly effective. Alternate heating and cooling methods (see page) are also most beneficial in osteo-arthritic disorders.

Application of Heated Needle

The needle is inserted to the required depth and then warmed with moxa in various forms.

1. *Moxa punk.* A piece of moxa punk is wrapped around the handle and ignited. When using this procedure it is advisable to place a piece of guard-paper around the base of the needle to catch any hot fragments which might fall (see Figure 14).
2. *Moxa slices.* A piece of moxa roll 1½-2cms (¾ in) long is cut off and a small hole pressed through its centre to enable it to be placed on the handle of the needle. Ready-made moxa plugs, suitable for placing on the handle of the needle, are available from Japan (Figure 15).

3. *Fire Needle caps.* These are small metal caps, designed to hold moxa punk, which fit over the handle of the needle. Because of their weight they are only suitable for needles with finer handles and of a thicker gauge (Figure 16).
4. *Moxa roll.* The glowing end of a moxa roll is held close to the point at the base of the needle until sufficient heat is attained (Figure 17). This is repeated in the usual manner of moxa roll technique. This is the most convenient method and is valuable in chronic conditions where an alternating stimulation and sedation technique is required.

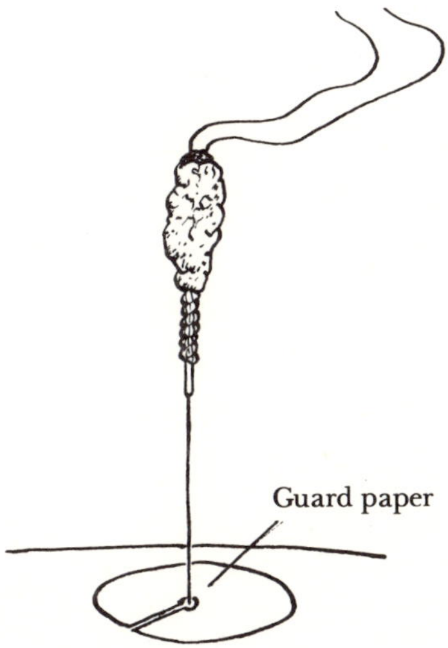

Figure 14. Heated needle technique with moxa punk.

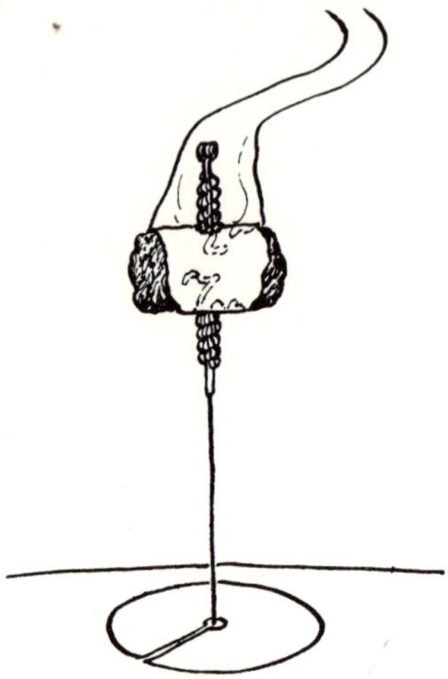

Figure 15. Heated needle technique with ready-made moxa plug.

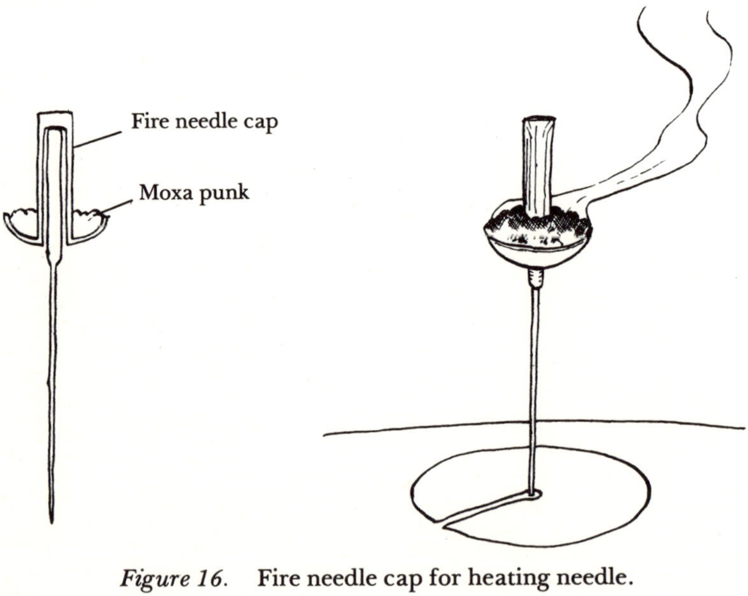

Figure 16. Fire needle cap for heating needle.

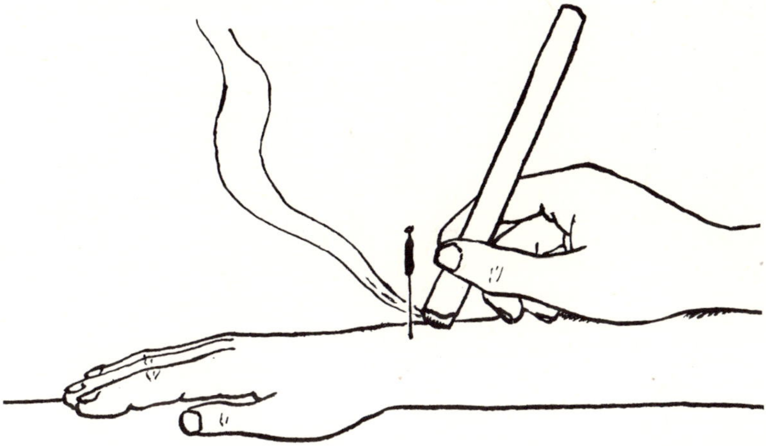

Figure 17. Heated needle technique with moxa roll.

REFERENCES

[1] Yi Shon Ji Jian, quoted in Lee, J. F. and Cheung, C. S., *Current Acupuncture Therapy* (Medical Book Publications, Hong Kong, 1978).
[2] Lee, J. F., and Cheung C. S., *op. cit.*

4

THE EFFECTS OF MOXIBUSTION

Centuries of effective use in the alleviation of man's ailments have failed to bring us much closer to a precise rationale for the mechanism of moxibustion. Current neuro-physiological research is beginning to provide some answers to certain aspects of the acupuncture and moxibustion phenomenon. Neurohumoral theories, for example, open a very promising avenue of research, but their plausibility should not blind us to the other unsolved problems that acupuncture poses, such as the specificity of points.

In arriving at a physiological basis for moxibustion we must consider its effects both in physical and metaphysical terms. The benefits it achieves undoubtedly operate at various levels, and in the final analysis it may be unnecessary to draw a distinction between them. As Porkert[1] states, 'We should always keep in mind that Western science is not more rational than Chinese science, merely more analytical.' Terminology and concepts may be different, but we may only be approaching the common solution from opposite directions.

In view of our present state of knowledge it is more suitable to consider physiological effects and traditional and energetic concepts separately.

Physiological Effects of Moxibustion

The main response to moxibustion is that of the body to any localized application of heat — initial vasoconstriction followed by vasodilatation. If the heat application is prolonged or repeated, as with direct moxibustion, or other strong stimulation technique, there is a release of histotoxins and a counter-irritant effect. Suppurative techniques make use of the heightened response and prolong the counter-irritation.

General Adaptation Syndrome

The principles of counter-irritation have been somewhat neglected in modern therapeutics. The mechanism is best understood in terms of Selye's concept of the General Adaptation Syndrome (G.A.S.). According to Selye[2] a general or local 'stressor' acting on the body initiates an 'alarm reaction' which, through excitation of the sympathetic nervous system and adrenal medulla, leads to a 'stage of resistance' as the body's defence mechanism begins to operate. There is a release of adrenal mineralocorticoids which localize the stressor and cause an inflammatory reaction, and of the glucocorticoid, cortisol, which has tissue-protective functions. Pain in any part of the body will generally precipitate an alarm reaction, but if prolonged, leads to the 'stage of exhaustion'. The initiation of a renewed G.A.S., by means of a target stressor at another site, reactivates the defensive mechanisms with a beneficial effect.

A general or local stimulation of the reticulo-endothelial system increases the immune response and may have correlations in energetic concepts with the idea of reinforcing the Wei-Chi.

Pain Control

In a consideration of the evolution of pain control, Toyama[3] has postulated three principles for the relief of pain. These are that alleviation will be achieved by:

1. Pressure at the centre of the pain.
2. Cold application at the centre of the pain.
3. Hot application at the centre of the pain.

Moxibustion can be placed in the third category whilst heated needle techniques belong in both (1) and (3): the pressure of the needle is combined with the localized application of heat.

The therapeutically optimal temperature is 70-80°C (158-176°F), but this would, in most cases of diffuse application, burn the skin. The greater the severity of the pain the higher the temperature required to alleviate it. Toyama has shown, however, that a small area of application minimizes the tendency to burn, whilst increasing heat production.[4] This is most effectively illustrated in the use of a piece of moxa the size of a rice grain which can attain the optimum heat without burning the skin.

Physiological Comparison of Cones and Rolls

The moxa cones are generally considered to have a deeper physiological effect than the rolls, although the latter are easier to use. An analogy would be the difference between radiant heat and infra-red. This produces an apparent contradiction since it is the shorter wave-lengths of infra-red which penetrate most deeply and, therefore, an incandescent source, which produces more of these than does a black body element, will produce a deeper penetration into the tissues.

By this principle, the glowing tip of a moxa roll should produce a deeper penetration than the pure heat of a cone, but in practice it appears that the cone tends to produce an effect before the patient feels any sense of discomfort and there is little erythema, whilst the roll produces a sharper feeling altogether, with marked erythema.

The roll naturally covers a wider area than the taper or greenstick, which appears to have a still sharper effect and less depth of penetration.

General Physiological Effects

The clinical observations of other workers have led to various conclusions as to the precise effects of moxibustion. The Cooperative Research Group of Moxibustion of Jianxi Province, China, recorded various physiological parameters during and after treatment of Chihyin, Bl 67, in cases of abnormal foetal position.[5] They noted that respiratory activity did not change significantly; superficial blood vessels dilated; pulse rate remained normal; systolic and diastolic pressure remained normal; differential count remained normal. These observations suggest that the sympathico-adrenal system was not stimulated by moxibustion, although a significant increase in the activity of the uterus was recorded.

A hormonal mechanism was suggested, however, by pre- and post-moxibustion measurements of 17-hydroxycorticosterone and 17-ketosteroids. Both hormones were found to be higher in pregnant women than in non-pregnant women and moxibustion increased the level of these still further in pregnant women. Pre-

and post-moxibustion determination of plasma corticosterone revealed similar variations. These results suggest that moxibustion stimulates the hypophyseal adreno-cortical system.

Point Specificity

Physicians at the Internal Peace Maternity and Child Health Hospital, China Welfare Institute, suggested a relative channel and point specificity in the treatment of abnormal foetal position.[6] Although Chihyin, Bl 67 point achieves an effective rate of 95.42 per cent, the moxibustion of Shaoshang, Lu.11, was totally ineffective in converting to vertex presentation.

A satisfactory physiological explanation for point specificity still remains to be determined, but clinical experience strongly suggests that it operates and that the traditional concept of meridian correlation to particular body tissues and functions has a firm basis.

Fumigation Effect

The ancient practice of burning moxa as an insecticide has been validated by later research. According to Fu Wei-kang, 'The aroma given off by burning moxa has been determined by modern science to be due to the volatile oil content of its leaves which is effective against certain disease producing bacteria.'[7]

Traditional and Energetic Concepts of Moxibustion

The foundation of acupuncture and moxibustion is the Tsang-Fu (Yin-Yang) theory. The effects of moxibustion have always been expressed in terms of its reinforcing and Yang nourishing properties. The warming and drying qualities of moxa drive out the 'perverse influences' of cold and damp.

The ancient text of *Ben Tsao Chong Sing*[8] states that moxa:

> . . . produces the warm ripe heat of the pure nature of Yang, [is] able to receive the critical stage of Yang, drain open the twelve meridians, enter into the three Yin, regulate air and blood, expel cold and wetness, warm the uterus, . . . used as a cauterizing fire it is able to permeate and penetrate into all meridians and rid various diseases.

The *Sou Wen* makes reference to the regional use of moxa in areas where cold and damp give rise to symptoms (see page 50). In a Materia Medica compiled by a distinguished medical scientist Li Shih-Chen (1518-93) it states that moxibustion has the effect of driving away cold and damp.

Forms of Energy

According to Porkert, Chinese medicine describes more than a dozen basic forms of energy and over two dozen accessory forms. These are, in many cases, different manifestations of the same force which may have bioelectric correlations in western physiology.

Porkert draws a useful analogy between Chinese terminology and that of electrical engineering.

> A legitimate—and from an epistemological point of view instructive—comparison is between the multiform terminology of Chinese energetics and the no less diversified terminology of electrical engineering in which expressions such as direct current, alternating current, light current, heavy current, high tensions, low tension, anode current, collector current, grid tension, high frequency, low frequency, and so on, always designate one basic phenomenon, electrical energy, which each term describes in regard to only one single, narrowly defined, empirical (technical) aspect which in ordinary usage is not specified. Exactly the same principle applies to the qualitatively rather than quantitatively differentiated energetic terminology in Chinese practical medicine.[9]

The different forms of Chi described by the ancient Chinese are merely various actions of the body in response to the fundamental energy. Energy probably has one basic form and is indivisible in terms of its kinetic or potential existence, although it may be convenient to conceptualize its various functional effects by a terminology of sub-division. The scientific validation of these concepts may, indeed, be a long way off. The life energies are such intangible forces that the very process of investigation alters their state. As Rose-Neil points out:

> All forms of present day science investigate by interference with function, by definition self-defeating in relation to energy.
>
> The necessary interference is difficult enough when investigating ordinary chemical phenomena, but at least chemicals have form, weight, and mass. But energy is weightless, massless, formless, as far as we know. Were it to take on a shape and mass, it would no longer be true energy.[10]

The acknowledgement that matter is capable of transmutation and, by implication, of differing effects upon its milieu, has come in the work of the French biochemist, Kervran.[11] He was able to demonstrate that living organisms are capable of synthesizing certain basic elements from others of different molecular structure. The concept of a Chi capable of transformation to perform different functions therefore has some foundation.

Defensive Energy

It is, for the moment, useful to recognize the transition between the Wei Chi, diffused throughout the body tissues, and Yong Chi, present in the meridians, often defined as two separate forms of energy but really only phases in the action of basic Chi. Wei Chi is regarded as the impure form of energy, particularly important as the first line of defence to the main meridians. It is the energy of the Tendino-muscular and Distinct meridians. The quality of the Wei energy governs the resistance of the body to the perverse influences of cold and damp — the 'External Devils'. Moxibustion reinforces this defensive action.

Stimulation and sedation techniques with heated needles are of value in dispersing the perverse influences of this nature, combining the reinforcement of defensive energy with the opening or loosening effect of the needle.

Perverse influences, however, often penetrate more deeply through the meridians, an effect attributed to an insufficiency of the 'purer' form of energy in the channels (Yong Chi). Once at this level there is greater likelihood of these influences having an adverse effect upon the organs and entrails. Over-enthusiastic needling of superficial disturbances of recent origin would tend to allow perverse energy into the meridian.

However nebulous the concept of Chi and its qualities of Yin and Yang may be, it provides the most satisfactory rationale for the therapeutic use and benefits of moxibustion. The application of traditional diagnostic principles also provides a more broadly-based foundation for the selection of the appropriate treatment than a purely empirical assessment.

A physician of the Emperor Jin, in 581 B.C., referred to the deep penetration of his patients' disease so that it could be neither 'attacked nor reached'. In the Han and Jin dynasties, 'attack' meant treatment by moxibustion and 'reach' meant treatment by acupuncture. The terms convey a nice distinction between the effects of the two forms of treatment and to sum up the benefits of moxibustion, we could borrow the military principle that 'attack is the best form of defence'.

REFERENCES

[1]Porkert, M., *Theoretical Foundations of Chinese Medicine* (M.I.T. Press, Cambridge, Mass. 1974).
[2]Selye, H., *Physiology and Pathology of Exposure to Stress* (Acta Inc., Montreal, 1950).
[3]Toyama, P. M., 'The Physiological Basis of Acupuncture and Moxibustion Therapy'. *American Journal of Acupuncture*, 3:2, 116, 1975).
[4]Toyama, P. M., *op. cit.*, p. 121.
[5]Co-operative Research Group of Moxibustion version of Jianxi Province, 'Clinical Investigation and Experimental Observations on Version by means of Moxibustion applied to Zhiyin points'. *Proc. Nat. Symposia of Acupuncture, Moxibustion, and Acupuncture Anaesthesia* (Beijing, 1979).
[6]Internal Peace Maternity and Child Health Hospital, 'Conversion of Breech Presentation by Moxibustion Fumigation of Zhiyin point'. *Proc. Nat. Symposia of Acupuncture, Moxibustion, and Acupuncture Anaesthesia* (Beijing, 1979).
[7]Fu Wei-kang, *The Story of Chinese Acupuncture and Moxibustion* (Foreign Languages Press, Peking, 1975).
[8]Ben Tsao Chong Sing, quoted in Cheung, C.S. and Lee, J. F., *op. cit.*
[9]Porkert, N., *op. cit.*, p. 167.
[10]Rose-Neil, S., *Acupuncture and The Life Energies* (British Acupuncture Association, London 1979).
[11]Kervran, C. L., *Biological Transmutations* (Crosby Lockwood, London, 1972).

5

DIAGNOSTIC ASSESSMENT

If moxibustion is to be used solely for its counter-irritant effects, diagnostic assessment becomes purely a matter of deciding upon the locality for the application. The use of diagnostic principles based on traditional concepts, however, considerably widens the scope of treatment and creates the need for a more precise rationale for the selection of the appropriate therapeutic regime.

The use of moxa without a consideration of the many possible variations in the equilibrium of Yin/Yang balance limits the potential value of the treatment. Since moxa has the properties of supplying energy and 'nourishing the Yang', a consideration of the patient's condition in these terms becomes imperative. The following survey of diagnostic methods is given primarily with reference to moxibustion and is designed to provide an orientation of thought rather than a detailed survey of the procedures. For more complete consideration of the various methods of diagnosis the practitioner should consult some of the excellent texts available.[1 2 3 4]

Broadly speaking, moxibustion has been considered by many as being more suitable for chronic disorders whilst needles were used in acute ailments, but, in energetic terms, moxa is essentially for diseases which exhibit the following (see also Figure 18):

- Yin excess with Yang deficiency
- Yin deficiency with Yang deficiency
- Yin normal with Yang deficiency
- Yin excess with Yang normal

It is, therefore, of greatest value for diseases due to cold, damp, and humidity; those in which there is flaccidity; those with spasm when due to excess Yin; and those due to emptiness of Yang.

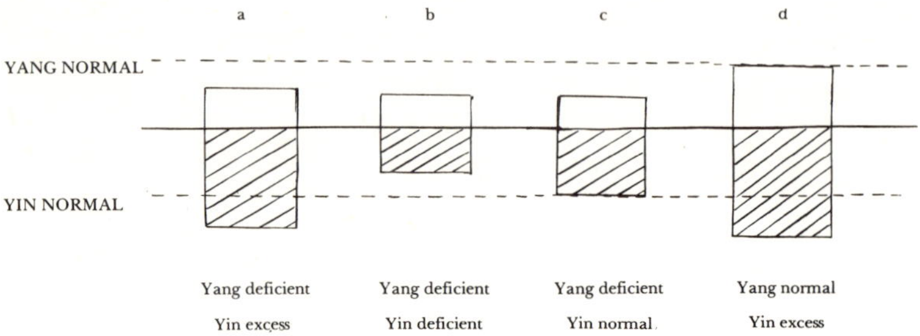

Figure 18. Energetic balance in conditions requiring moxibustion.

In selecting the most appropriate treatment, it is necessary to determine the state of the blood and Chi and the equilibrium of Yin and Yang. Utilizing the traditional methods of seeing, hearing, asking, feeling, and pulse diagnosis, the real nature of the complaint may be determined by application of the Eight Diagnostic Rules.

The Eight Diagnostic Rules

These provide a systematic framework for the assessment of the quality, nature, and depth of the patient's disorder. The Eight Principles or Diagnostic Rules are:

- Yin and Yang (Tsang and Fu)
- Cold and Hot (Han and Re)
- Emptiness and Fullness (Xu and Ji)
- Internal and External (Li and Piao)

These are all features of the patient's ailments which can be distinguished, although apparently contradictory qualities may be the chief features of the condition, e.g., emptiness of Yang (Yang-Xu) in chronic diarrhoea.

Since a clear understanding of these features is essential to the practice of moxibustion, we shall briefly consider each pair of qualities.

Yin and Yang (Tsang-Fu)

These are the two main principles which distinguish the different groups of disorders. They are very broad categories which embrace the other six diagnostic principles. Assessment of Yin/Yang quality helps to determine the development of the illness and its localization.

Ailments which are localized in the surface tissues, secondary vessels and principal meridians, are generally Yang, whilst those involving the organs and entrails are Yin. We should, however, guard against the tendency to classify diseases as Yin or Yang purely on their location as superficial or deep, or because they involve Yin or Yang organs. Yin organs may frequently have Yang diseases for which moxibustion would be contra-indicated, e.g., a condition of dry heat in the liver in a cirrhotic disorder.

The main distinguishing features of Yin disorders are as follows:

— The symptoms tend to move inwards
— Tendency to withdraw, little talking, lying curled up
— Respiration feeble
— Seeks warmth, no thirst, urine clear
— Limbs cold
— Pulse deep and slow
— Tongue pale, moist, indented (teeth marks)

The Yang qualities of movement to the surface, and upper part of the body, seeking coldness, thirst for cold drinks, pulse full, hard, or bounding, and tongue dry and coated, are generally, though not absolutely, contra-indications to moxibustion. This may depend upon consideration of the localization of the malady.

Cold and Hot (Han-Re)

This indicates the state of the disease. If the patient fears the cold and craves warmth, and the body is cold, a disorder is classed as a 'cold', Yin type, 'deficiency' disease. The converse is true of Yang disorders.

There are frequently manifestations of both hot and cold in the body, or parts of it, and before selecting treatment it is necessary to determine whether one is confronted with combinations of hot and cold, or localization of heat or coolness in the upper or lower parts of the body, or a reciprocal variation of hot and cold within one area.

Clinical signs of cold disorders may include:

— No thirst
— Limbs cold
— Pale skin
— Urine abundant and clear
— Tongue whitish
— Pulse slow

The clinical signs of coldness in the upper part of the body are:

— Breathlessness
— Indigestion
— Vomiting

Coldness in the lower part of the body manifests as:

— Stools hard and dry
— Abdominal pain
— Herniation
— Limbs cold

More complex interactions with other couples occur when perverse influences move within the body. According to the *Sou Wen* (Chapter 5):

> Cold, with fullness, moves down and transforms to heat; the heat, with fullness, moves upwards and transforms to cold.

The symptom complexes which arise in these circumstances can give a false impression of Yin/Yang equilibrium. They are generally referred to as conditions of 'false Yang', causing symptoms such as restlessness, constipation, dyspnoea, painful throat, and thirst without desire to drink.

In the presence of signs of general weakness, quiet voice, pale clear urine, tongue flabby and coated at the centre, pulse deep, fine, and feeble, the disorder may be due to the presence of cold perverse energy calling for moxibustion reinforcement.

Emptiness and Fullness (Xu-Ji)

This determines the state of the essential energy of the body in relation to the perverse energy. If there is insufficient body energy (emptiness), the perverse energy is able to penetrate the organism.

In general, 'fullness', and 'emptiness', can be distinguished by palpation of the affected areas. In emptiness (deficiency of Yang) firm pressure is comforting and gives relief (by increasing the compressive qualities of Yang). In fullness (excess Yang) pressure aggravates the discomfort (by adding to the excess).

According to the *Sou Wen* (Chapter 28):

> Perverse energy is a strong energy which engenders fullness. The energy of the body, when attacked by the perverse energy is enfeebled and becomes empty.

Nguyen Van Nghi,[1] therefore, proposes the following rules:

1. The energy of the body in a state of weakness = emptiness.
2. Empty energy of the body + perverse energy = fullness.

In assessing the requirements of the patient it is necessary to discover the cause of the fullness or emptiness, its localization in the blood, and to distinguish between the true and false manifestations of these qualities.

The signs of emptiness are:

— Fine pulse

— Cold skin

— Weakness

— Diarrhoea

— Abundant urine

In general the constitution of the patient is a good indication of fullness and emptiness. Those of slender and feeble constitution tend to suffer from the disorders of emptiness which require reinforcement.

A distinction needs to be made between the relative states of the tendino-muscular and principal meridians. In the *Sou Wen* the following advice is given:

> When the tendino-muscular meridian is full and the principal meridian is empty, it is necessary to moxa the principal meridian and puncture the tendino-muscular meridian.

When the tendino-muscular meridian is empty and the principal meridian is full, it is necessary to moxa the tendino-muscular and puncture the principal meridian.

Fullness of the tendino-muscular meridian will manifest as spasms and contractions with acute sensitivity of superficial points. Pulse diagnosis may reveal a relative deficiency of the principal meridian. In this situation the tendino-muscular meridian should be punctured on painful points and the tonification point of the principal meridian is given moxibustion.

Emptiness of tendino-muscular meridians may be evidenced by weakness, numbness, and flaccidity. There will be tenderness on deep palpation, though not a sharp sensitivity to superficial touch. If this is accompanied by fullness of the corresponding principal meridian, its sedation point should be punctured, whilst moxa may be applied to local points of the tendino-muscular meridian. (Some authorities recommend that, in either case, the action on the principal meridian should be taken at the Tsing point).

Internal and External (Li-Piao)
These qualities designate the locality of the malady and overlap aspects of the other diagnostic principles. Their significance in terms of moxibustion depends upon the nature of the perverse energy which has caused the ailment. Disorders due to cold may require moxa treatment, whether they manifest in the external zone (epidermis, principal meridians, and secondary vessels) or internally (organs and entrails), although it is more likely to be of value in the former.

The symptomatology of external disorders, due to the invasion of cold, includes: headaches, radiating from the neck; fear of cold; pains in the joints; tongue thin and whitish; pulse superficial and fast. The pulse of external disorders due to emptiness of Yang is superficial and slow.

Internal disorders due to cold manifest as symptoms which include: cold limbs; lack of perspiration; abdominal pains; nausea and vomiting; tongue coated and moist; pulse deep and rapid. Emptiness of Yang Chi internally gives rise to feeble respiration, poor appetite, cold limbs, tachycardia, tongue whitish, pulse deep and very fine.

The symptomatology may be complicated by the fact that

manifestations of disorders at both external and internal levels may appear.

Perverse Energies

In the overall diagnostic assessment of a patient's condition the analysis of the interaction of the Eight Principles must also be modified by a consideration of the influence of the perverse energies.

The term 'perverse energy' is applied to any otherwise normal exogenous or endogenous phenomenon which creates a disturbance because of disequilibrium in the body's function. Ailments most commonly arise from failure to adjust to climatic factors which create disturbances in the external zones, and initially in the Tai Yang meridian (Si, Bl). Moxa should be used where indicated to reinforce the defensive energy.

Of the exogenous perverse energies, or 'External Devils' — wind (Fong), cold (Han), heat (Shu), humidity (Shih), dryness (Zao), fire (Huo) — the wind, cold, and humidity, or their combined effects, are most likely to call for moxibustion. Each of the perverse energies has its own predominant symptomatology which has been outlined in relation to the diagnostic principles. The internal perverse energies, such as fear, anger, depression, may create disturbances when the equilibrium of the meridians, by which they are controlled, is disturbed. Moxibustion may also be of value in reinforcing the Yang energy of these where there is such an instability.

There are many aetiological permutations of the perverse influences and the diagnostic principles and they can be interpreted in terms of a number of different aspects of Chinese physiology, not least of which are the Law of Five Elements and the Eight Extra Meridians.

Law of Five Elements

The concept of the Five Elements, more suitably termed the 'Five Transformations',[5] relates to the movement of energy in the outer layers; the interaction of the body with its immediate environment.[6] Disturbance of equilibrium within the cycle may create a susceptibility to perverse influences.

The above diagnostic criteria may be used to determine disturbances of individual meridians within the cycle. A deficiency of any meridian, for example the Lung, would affect the equilibrium of the whole system by the Sheng, Ko, and Mo cycles. There would, in the case of lung deficiency, be a secondary deficit of kidney energy and a relative excess of the liver. This is not, however, an excess upon which to draw and the correct course of action is to supply the Lung meridian, which may be done by moxibustion to the source point (Lu 9) and or the Associated Effect (Back Shu) points (Bl 13).

Moxibustion is, therefore, of value in rebalancing the Five Transformations, on the basis of meridian symptomatology and, particularly, when there is insufficient energy elsewhere in the cycle upon which to draw.

Eight Extra Meridians—The Irregular Vessels

A general deficiency of energy in the channels may indicate a need for the use of the Irregular Vessels, particularly the Yin Wei/Chong Mo and Yin Keo/Ren Mo couples.

Yin Wei/Chong Mo are associated with organic insufficiencies, in particular those in which ancestral energy (Yuan Chi) is poor. The Key points of this couple, Neikuan, HC 6, and Kungsun, Sp 4, are amenable to moxibustion. Yin Keo/Ren Mo are implicated in conditions of female Yin, particularly those associated with disturbance of fluid metabolism. Fluid retention problems are treated by needling or moxa to the key points Chaohai, Ki 6, and Liehchueh, Lu 7, and applying moxa to Shuifen, VC 9.

Conclusion

Diagnosis consists of a series of investigations and assessments in terms of the above-mentioned criteria. The therapeutic regime may be built up using as its framework one or more of these phenomena, depending on the complexity of the complaint. To this basic framework must be brought the specialized knowledge, accumulated over many generations, which is the foundation of a well-tried treatment repertory.

There are also some clinical situations which require special consideration.

REFERENCES

[1]Nguyen Van Nghi, *Pathogénie et Pathologie Energetiques en Médicine Chinoise* (Imprimerie Ecole Technique Don Bosco, Marseilles, 1971).
[2]Chamfrault, A. and Nguyen Van Nghi, *L'Énergetiques Humaine en Médicine Chinoise*. Vol. 4 of *Traité de Médicine Chinoise* (Imprimerie de la Charante, Angouleme 1969).
[3]Woollerton, H. and McLean, C. J., *Acupuncture Energy in Health and Disease* (Thorsons Publishers, Wellingborough, 1979).
[4]Deadman, P., 'Differentiation of Disease according to the Eight Conditions', *Journal of Chinese Medicine*, Nos. 4, and 5, 1980.
[5]Porkert, M. *Theoretical Foundations of Chinese Medicine*, *op. cit.*
[6]Rausenberger, P. 'Movement of Energy', Third Korth Lecture. British Acupuncture Association Congress, London, 1980.

6

THERAPEUTIC CONSIDERATIONS AND CLINICAL DATA

One must always remember the basic rule that 'needles transfer the energy, moxa puts energy in'. This does not imply that moxa may not be used as a stimulus for energy transference, for many of its benefits are undoubtedly the result of this process. There are, however, some other clinical considerations which may prove valuable in selecting the most suitable points and mode of application, particularly in the management of combined symptoms due to both hot and cold, or internal and external factors.

Selecting Points and Mode of Application

The guidance offered by the ancient texts prove as valuable as any. The following passage from the *Sou Wen* (Chapter 60) gives guidelines in the use of moxibustion.

> The method of applying moxibustion to treat cold-hot symptoms is such that the Tachui point (Gv 14) in the back of the neck should be treated first, and the number of moxa-sticks to be applied should be determined by the patient's age; then, the coccyx point should be treated by moxibustion and the number of moxa-sticks to be applied should be determined by the patient's age. Apply moxibustion to the depressed spots at the edge of the clavicle; apply moxibustion to the depression while the patient is lifting up his arm and shoulder (i.e., Chienyu, Co 15); apply moxibustion to the points between the two ribs region (Chingmen, GB 25); apply moxibustion to the tip of the depression just above the lateral malleolus (Yangfu, GB 38); apply moxibustion to the point in between the little toe and the fourth toe

(Hsiahsi, GB 43); apply moxibustion to the depression below the calf (Chengchin, Bl 56); apply moxibustion to the region above the supraclavicular fossa where pain and hardness occur like tendons; apply moxibustion to the depression in the pectoralis major region (Tientu, VC 22); apply moxibustion to the region below the head of the ulna (Yangchih, TH 4); apply moxibustion to the Kuanyuan point (VC 4) three osteo units below the navel; apply moxibustion to the artery at the edge of the pubic hair (Chichung, St 30); apply moxibustion to the region in between tendons and three osteo units below the knee (Tsusanli, St 36); apply moxibustion to the arteries on the back of the foot on the Bright Yang of foot meridian (Chungyang, St 42); apply moxibustion to the top of the head (Paihui, GV 20); apply moxibustion in the amount of three sticks of moxa to the dog-bite, because dog-bite will also cause cold and hot sensations; thus, there are a total of twenty-nine places where moxibustion may be applied. Injuries caused by consumption of foods may also be treated by moxibustion, but if it does not recover by moxibustion, apply acupuncture for many times to the points on the meridian displaying Yang excess which has become visible, and then apply herbal therapy.[1]

Cones or Rolls

The use of the moxa cone is most called for over the Shu points (Associated Effect Points), and over special points, such as Shuifen, VC 9, which is a main point for control of body fluid. The roll is quicker and more convenient, but it is the opinion of the authors that the cone gives better results. Bearing in mind the old statement that 'the kidneys rule the bones', a very good example would be in the use of fairly strong moxibustion on Shenshu, Bl 23 and Chihshih, Bl 47 in all cases where bones are affected, i.e., as supportive treatment in all arthritic conditions, but especially in such cases as Osgood-Schlatter's Disease, osteoporosis, osteomalacia, even osteomyelitis, or in the use of moxa over Chaohai, Ki 6, Liehchueh, Lu 7 and Shuifen, VC 9 for fluid retention, and similar cases.

The roll is particularly useful where a large area is to be covered with a constant, gentle heating for possibly four to five minutes, as in its use for helping to soften scar-tissue, and also for heating around the needle.

Heated Needles

This latter technique is of particular interest for, although the effect of moxa in general is stimulatory, we would suggest that in heating around a needle which is placed in for dispersal, the moxa actually increases the dispersal effect, most probably by the increase in local erythema around the needle with a counter-irritant effect, similar to a topical rubefacient, but which, in traditional terminology, would be regarded as a summoning of abherrant energy for dispersal via the capillary network. It is interesting to note that this technique has been found, in practice, to be more effective when used over points of the Tai Yang meridian (Si, Bl) which is not only the most superficial of the channels, but which is regarded as possessing more blood than energy.

This supply and dispersal technique may be the reason for the success of heated needles in the management of back pain due to degenerative disc lesions or hypotonia. One of the authors (R.N.T.) has found this procedure particularly effective in such disorders and has postulated a tissue protective function via the Back Shu points of related organs, such as the liver and kidneys.[2]

Periodic Heating Technique

This heated needle technique is used most specifically for osteo-arthritic conditions. A needle is placed into the selected point to the required depth, and left in situ. After five minutes a piece of moxa punk is wrapped around the handle and ignited. The punk should be of such a size that it burns for two minutes, after which it is left to cool down for a further three minutes, making a total of five minutes in all. The ash is now carefully removed, a further piece of punk wrapped round and ignited, and after five minutes the process is repeated. After the third piece of punk has been burnt through and the needle has cooled, the ash is removed and the needle taken out, the whole cycle thus having taken a total of twenty minutes.

Minutes	*Needle*
0	Insert
5	Heat
10	Heat
15	Heat
20	Withdraw

(It is possible to heat the handle with a match, lighter, etc., for about thirty seconds until at least red-hot, but it has been found that moxa punk gives just the right temperature for the optimum effect.)

The reason for this rather specific technique is that osteoarthrosis, particularly if it is fairly advanced, can be regarded as a mixed Yin and Yang condition. Yin, logically, because it is cold and chronic, and Yang in that there is pain and possibly spasm in the area. So we use a mixed Yin/Yang treatment, with dispersal, to help relax, and heat to stimulate the local circulation and to help 'loosen things up'. This description of its action has been of a rather over-simplified Western approach, but it does give an easily understood mental picture of what it actually does.

The Great Points
It should be noted that this is a purely local treatment for a specific joint, and it has been found, through practice, that there are certain points which have a particularly effective action on their related joint when used in this manner. Some of these Chinese tradition has named as the 'Great Points' for rheumatic conditions, others have been found by one of the authors (Royston Low) in his own practice, and the point for each of the various joints likely to be affected are shown in Table 1.

Whilst dealing with arthritic conditions, there is a very interesting specific technique called for when there is a pain present in the acromioclavicular joint, and that is the use of what is termed 'blown' moxas. A large cone of punk (about the size of a hazelnut), is placed directly upon the acromial process, ignited, and then blown on to hasten the combustion. The process is repeated for a total of three moxas.

Gradual Warming Procedure
The next category of heated needle, wherein a piece of moxa roll, or moxa plug is placed over the handle, produces a completely different effect. In this case the heat is steady throughout and produces a strong, constant warmth. As in all cases of intervention into the biosphere of the body, a stimulus carried on over a certain length of time produces an opposite reaction to that produced by a short intervention, and here we find that the strong but steady heat produces an effect which is relaxing to the surrounding tissues, yet simultaneously stimulates the local flow of blood and lymph in the area. It is particularly effective when dealing with fibrositic nodules and localized spasmodic conditions. Whilst in Peking we noticed the great use made of this technique, especially when using Fengshih (GB 20) for headaches and migraine to relax

TABLE 1. THE GREAT POINTS FOR OSTEO-ARTHRITIC DISORDERS

Area	*Points*	*Remarks*
Mandibular joint	Hsiakuan (St 7)	Particularly effective for osteo-chondritis of this joint.
Occipital area	Fengfu (GV 16)	
Cervico-thoracic area	Taotao (GV 13)	Or, occasionally, Tachui (GV 14), though this latter should be used with care, as it is the meeting point of the upper Yang meridians and one must often balance its use with Tachu (Bl 11).
Thoracic area	Chihyang (GV 9)	
Lumbar area	Mingmen (GV 4)	
Shoulder	Chienyu (Co 15) Chupi (special point)	
Elbow	Chuchih (Co 11)	
Wrist	Yangchih (TH 4)	Or, occasionally, for osteo-arthrosis of the ulnar-styloid and pisiform area, Wanku (SI 4).
Thumb	Yanghsi (Co 5)	
Hip-joint	Huantiao (GB 30)	
Knee	Weiyang (Bl 53) Hsihsia (special point)	
Ankle	Chiehhsi (St 41) Chungyang (St 42)	
Hallux joint	Chihping (special point)	Not heated needle, but seven moxas.

the associated tension in the trapezius and longissimus capitis muscles. It is extremely effective in cases of sacro-iliac strain, where one selects from either Kuanyuanshu (Bl 26) or an Ahshi point between Bl 26 and special point Yaoyi. In some cases of arthritis of the metacarpal joint of the thumb, where Yangshi (Co 5) has been 'tried and found wanting', this technique applied to Taiyuan (Lu 9) has been found effective.

It is, naturally, to be understood that these specific points with heated needles are supplemented with ordinary acupuncture procedures in all the conditions described.

Treatment of Paralysis
A differentiation needs to be made between paralysis due to upper and lower motor-neuron lesions since the energetic interpretation of spastic and flaccid paralysis differs (see Figure 19).

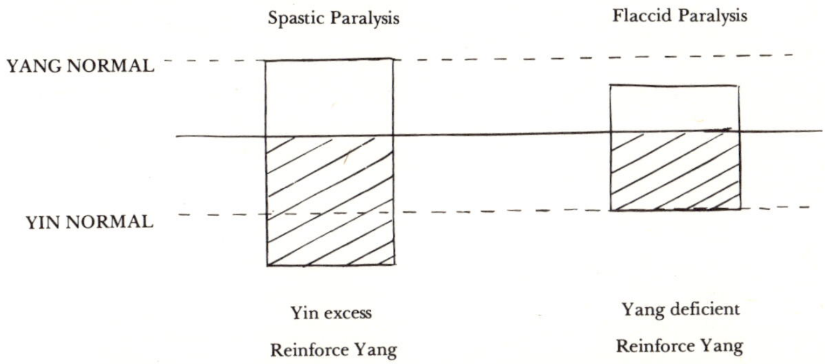

Figure 19. Energetic action of moxibustion in paralysis.

In flaccid paralysis there is a deficit of Yang, so ordinary moxa treatment will suffice to bring this up to balance the Yin. With spastic paralysis, however, there is normal Yang with an excess of Yin. The Yin cannot be drained so the Yang must be reinforced to meet it, and this can best be achieved by inserting the needle in the appropriate point (especially Yanglingshuan, Gb 34), heating the needle with a spirit lamp until red hot and withdrawing the needle whilst it is still glowing—not with bare fingers!

Clinical Data

Research workers throughout the world, and particularly in China, have accumulated a considerable amount of evidence as to the benefits of moxibustion. We do not propose to reduplicate data which merely corroborates the efficacy of a treatment which has proved its worth over many hundreds of years, but it is interesting to note its value in disorders which might not be considered amenable to moxibustion, or may even be considered to be contra-indications on the basis of Tsang-Fu theory. The following reports are summarized to indicate the wide scope of moxibustion.

Hypertension

Chen Daizhong, et al,[3] have shown that scarring moxibustion, by lowering the viscosity of blood and dilating blood vessels, is effective in the prevention and the treatment of hypertension. In observations on fifty-four cases of hypertension over a period of seventeen years, only five showed cardio-vascular accidents, compared with a control group of twelve patients in whom four had C.V.A.'s.

Facial Paralysis

Various authors have reported success in the use of combined needle and moxa therapy for facial paralysis. At the Department of Acupuncture and Moxa of Chong Chun Institute of Traditional Chinese Medicine, 1,008 cases of facial paralysis were treated with 'local moxibustion to promote perspiration, by needling every other day with prismatic needles, and letting of blood of the cheek on the diseased side into the aural cavity, then by acupuncture as an auxilliary measure to Hegu (Co 4) and Tsusanli (St 36)'. They reported a complete cure of 61 per cent of the total with an overall success rate of 96 per cent.[4]

Shao Jinming,[5] of the Honan College of Traditional Chinese Medicine, reporting on combined treatments for facial paralysis, states that 'if the effect of acupuncture is not obvious the moxibustion should be added to the points Dicang (St 4) and Jiachi (St 6) in order to warm the channels, exclude the cold, and restore the physiological function.' The author also forbids washing with cold water and advises a mask to protect against the cold. Complete recovery was achieved in 75 per cent of cases with 'excellent' response in a further 15 per cent.

Asthma

Regular treatment with suppurative moxibustion in 299 cases treated at the Department of Acupuncture of Yueyang Hospital,

Shanghai College of Traditional Chinese Medicine, achieved beneficial effects in over 70 per cent according to Yen Hua.[6] All cases were treated in summer time on points Dazhu (Bl 11), and Feishu (Bl 13), to which moxa was applied three times every other day.

An improvement was also observed in the haemoglobin and red blood cell count of patients undergoing treatment.

Breech Presentation of Foetus

The application of moxibustion to Zhiyin (Bl 67) in the treatment of breech presentation has been widely reported. Wang Wenshih[7] of the Fourth People's Hospital, Shenyang applied treatment for 15 minutes once daily for a few days on 2,069 cases with a success rate of 90.32 per cent. According to Wenshih, abnormal position results from a loss of equilibrium between bladder and kidney channels.

Acute Lymphangitis

At the Gansu Hospital of Traditional Chinese Medicine, 138 cases of acute lymphangitis were treated between 1960 and 1972 using a heated needle technique with moxa sticks. Needles were placed near the malignant boil and in Ashi points at each end of the affected area. A spreading technique of moxibustion was used over the area for 15 to 20 minutes.

A 78.9 per cent success rate after one treatment was recorded with another 20 per cent recovering after a further one or two treatments.[8]

Hot Needling for Benign Swellings

Fernando and Jayasuriya[9] refer to the ancient 'hot needling' technique for various types of benign swelling, including goitres and ganglia. A Yuan-Li needle is heated to red or white heat, inserted rapidly, and immediately withdrawn, at various sites in the swelling.

Yuan-Li needling has been used by one of the authors (Royston Low) on numerous occasions and has been found to be extremely efficacious in cases of ganglia (particularly old, fibrosed ones which do not respond to the usual dispersal techniques), Baker's cysts of the popliteal fossa, and similar benign swellings.

The needle is heated to red/white heat over a spirit lamp and is plunged swiftly into the centre of the swelling (if large, several sites may be used) and immediately withdrawn. In some cases, two or three applications at about weekly intervals may be required. Strangely enough, all patients report that the treatment is not painful — certainly less so than needling the Tsing points!

REFERENCES

[1] *Sou Wen*, tr. Henry Lu (Academy of Oriental Heritage, Vancouver, B.C.).
[2] Newman Turner, R., 'The Role of Acupuncture in the Management of the Back Pain Syndrome', British Acupuncture Association Congress, Oxford, 1978.
[3] Chen Daizhong, Xu Yuzhan, and Tang Hong Zhi, 'A Clinical Investigation in the Prevention and Treatment of Hypertension by Scarring Moxibustion', *Proc. National Symposia of Acupuncture and Moxibustion and Acupuncture Anaesthesia*, p. 57, Beijing, 1979.
[4] Chang Chun Institute of Traditional Chinese Medicine, 'Analytical Report of the Therapeutic Effect of Acupuncture Treatment for Peripheral Facial Paralysis', *op. cit.*, p. 73.
[5] Shao Jin Ming, 'Treatment of Peripheral Facial Paralysis with Acupuncture and Moxibustion — An Observation of 60 cases', *op. cit.*, p. 75.
[6] Yen Hua, 'The Clinical Study of the Treatment of Asthma by Purulent Moxibustion', *op. cit.*, p. 58.
[7] Wang Wenshih, 'Clinical Analysis of Moxibustion in Correcting Abnormal Foetal Position', *op. cit.*, p. 93.
[8] Gansu Hospital of Traditional Chinese Medicine, 'A Clinical Observation of 138 cases of Acute Lymphangitis Treated with Acupuncture and Moxibustion', *op. cit.*, p. 99.
[9] Jayasuriya, A. and Fernando, F., *Principles and Practice of Scientific Acupuncture* (Lake House Investments Limited, Colombo, 1978).

7

THERAPEUTIC REPERTORY

The following repertory of clinical applications for moxibustion has been drawn up as a reference for acupuncture practitioners. The recommendations are based on the personal experience of the authors as well as being drawn from classical and modern texts. Only specially effective points or techniques have been included here. There will, of course, be other local points of value because of their proximity or energetic relationship to the tissues involved.

It must be re-emphasized that these techniques should only be used in the context of a total therapeutic regime based on the principles of acupuncture. Before treating any malady the patient's overall condition must be assessed and the appropriate treatment selected in terms of the diagnostic principles and rules of acupuncture.

TABLE 2. TREATMENT OF FORMULAS

Condition	*Moxa Treatment*	*Remarks and Rationale*
Respiratory General chest conditions including bronchitis and pneumonia	Straight line from Bl 37 across GV 12 to Bl 37 on opposite side.	Warm gently with spreading technique for 15-20 minutes.

Condition	*Moxa Treatment*	*Remarks and Rationale*
Chronic bronchitis	GV 14, Bl 12, Bl 13, VC 17	Moxa 3-5 x each.
Asthma	VC 21. Painful points in area of Bl 17.	
Asthma (of 'cold' nature)	Bl 13, VC 12, VC 17, Lu 7, Bl 38	Shu point of Lung.
Asthma (with productive cough)	VC 9	
Hiccough	VC 17 VC 12 VC 4	Upper heater, 5-9 x. Middle heater, 5-9 x. 5-9 x. Can add Bl 23.
Abdominal		
General abdominal pains	Special point on medial aspect of 1st metatarsal bone at level of Li 3, also Li 1, Li 2. Area at the root of great toe nail and outer corners of nail. Tip of spinous process of 3rd lumbar vertebra.	Simultaneously needle GV 4, Bl 25, Bl 27 (see below) 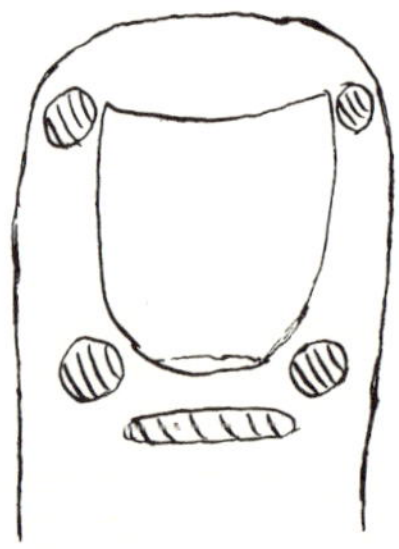 Great toe
Abdominal swelling	VC 6, Bl 20, Bl 17, Li 13	
Abdominal pain from mucus congestion	VC 14, VC 10, St 40	
Abdominal pain with loose stool and cold feet	VC 14, VC 4	
Acute indigestion	Tips of fingers and thumb of one hand (traditionally left for male and right for female).	Moxa once for each year of age to a maximum of 50 or warm until pain disappears.
Gastralgia	VC 12, St 36	Between attacks of pain.

Condition	*Moxa Treatment*	*Remarks and Rationale*
—gastralgia with cough	Warm circular area about 4cm (1½ ins) diameter directly below areola of each nipple.	Easiest with men. Treat for about 5-6 minutes.
Peptic ulcer	GV 8, Bl 17, Sp 8, GB 34	
Cirrhosis of liver	Bl 18	Shu point of liver.
Intestinal problems	Tip of olecranon of elbow and Co 11. If acute, heat along stomach lines from St 25 to St 27.	10-30 x. 6-8 minutes.
Diverticulitis	Special points: (a) between St 25 and St 26 and (b) between St 26 and St 27.	Compound treatment consisting of: needle St 25; moxa 5 x, special point (a); needle St 26; needle special point (b); moxa 5 x, St 27. (This treatment can be used in many bowel conditions with the needles either tonifying or draining, but moxas will balance whilst draining.)
Appendicitis	Special point level with spine of 3rd lumbar vertebra, 3 cun from mid-line on the right.	Moxa 40 x, then needle Bl 18.
Diarrhoea	St 25, VC 11. Special point Yaochi in the depression below the spinous process of the 2nd sacral vertebra.	Needle for epilepsy.
Chronic dysentery	VC 8, VC 12, St 25, VC 4, St 31, Bl 23.	

Condition	*Moxa Treatment*	*Remarks and Rationale*
Constipation	Special point (extension of Ki 16) between St 25 and Ki 16 at ½ cun inside St 25.	Moxa special point and Ki 16 bilaterally 7 x each. Can be augmented by 1 moxa, with a roll, at each corner of the open mouth. (Can alternate with Co 2.)
Constipation due to congestion of Yin.	VC 4, Sp 6.	Reunion points of lower Yin meridians.
Haemorrhoids	Yaochi (in depression below tip of 2nd sacral vertebra). GV 2. Special point caudal to GV 2 in notch of coccyx; GV 1. Special point anterior to GV 1 on rim of anus.	Moxa 20 x each. Recommend pecking technique, greenstick moxa —3 treatments at weekly intervals are usually sufficient.
Vomiting and hiatus hernia	Special points (a) between VC 14 and VC 15, (b) between VC 15 and VC 16, (c) and (d) on each side of VC 15 at 1 cun distance.	Treatment by moxa 5 times on each point (can include VC 15 if desired). (See below.) 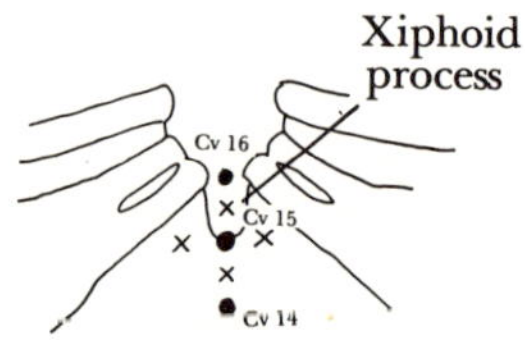
Worms	Special points close to the sternum between Ki and VC lines: (a) between 1st and 2nd ribs, (b) between 2nd and 3rd ribs.	These points used in specific manner; moxa 3 x first day, 5 x the second, 7 x the third, on all four points. Wait 3 days and repeat if necessary.
Circulatory Conditions Heart pains	Special point between TH 4 and Co 5 (Chungchuan).	Heat for 5 minutes.

Condition	*Moxa Treatment*	*Remarks and Rationale*
Poor circulation: —arms & hands —legs & feet	 Bl 11. St 37, St 39. Bl 32.	 Sea of Blood points. 21 x in rice-size cones.
Varicosities	Special points on palm, on the 'heart' line (transverse) below the prolongations of the 2nd and 3rd fingers.	Moxa 3 x bilaterally and add drainage needles to two special points 4 cun above the wrist crease medial and lateral to the HC meridian between the tendons.
Urinary Conditions All bladder problems	Tip of spinous process of 3rd lumbar vertebra and add Bl 28.	3-9 x.
Enuresis	GV 20, GV 4, VC 4, VC 12	2 or 3 points each treatment daily.
Incontinence	Special point below VC 2, immediately below the pubic bone.	Moxa 7 x with care
Fluid retention	Ki 6, Lu 7, VC 9, moxa special point and/or centre of the 1st phalanx of the 2nd toe.	Points of Yin Keo/Ren Mo, moxa 7 x.
Nephritis	Special point anterior to Sp 10 on the outer border of the sartorius muscle.	Moxa 7 x.
Urinary flow difficulties	Special point between Bl 62 and Bl 64.	Moxa 5 x.
Renal calculus	VC 7.	
Retention of urine	Bl 22, Bl 27, VC 3, Bl 67 or GV 28, Li 4, Li 3.	Can alternate formulas.

Condition	*Moxa Treatment*	*Remarks and Rationale*
Genital and Obstetric		
Female genital problems	(a) Sp 6, Chengming (1 cun posterior to Sp 6), (b) centre of the phalanx of the hallux and the area of the root of the nail.	Heat bilaterally for 6-8 minutes.
Dysmenorrhoea	Special point between Ki 3 and Ki 4, slightly posterior. Also Ki 3, Ki 5 and heat around the tip of the medial malleolus. VC 4, VC 2, Tzukung (3 cun beside VC 3).	Moxa 10 x. Can add the Bafeng points between the toes (traditionally, as only for women, use the right side). Heat 10-20 minutes.
Menses		
—late from deficiency of blood.	Sp 6, Sp 10, VC 6, St 28.	Add drainage needle to VC 3.
—excessive	(a) dorsum of 5th toe. (b) root of big toe nail.	6-8 minutes. 2 minutes.
—irregular	VC 4.	3-5 x on ginger, after the period, every other day for 10 treatments.
Functional uterine haemorrhage	(a) Sp 6, Bl 20, Bl 18, Sp 1 and points from (b) GV 4, VC 4, Sp 10, Li 10, GV 20.	Select from 1-3 points from (a) and moxa 5-7 x daily. If the condition is of a Xu (deficient) nature add GV 4 and VC 4. If of a Ji (full) nature add Sp 10 and Li 1. If there is very severe bleeding add GV 20.
Uterine haemorrhage	Li 1.	Moxa 7 x.
Haemorrhage after abortion	Li 1.	Moxa 3 x.
Uterine prolapse	VC 6, Sp 6.	Heat with stick 10-15 minutes.
Retroversion of uterus	Tip of spinous process of 5th lumbar vertebra.	Heat for 5 minutes. Also needle VC 3.

Condition	*Moxa Treatment*	*Remarks and Rationale*
Frigidity impotence (either sex)	Special points bilaterally, ½ cun from mid-line and ¼ cun above level of VC 7.	Moxa each point 5 x and needle VC 7.
	Can add further special point 6 cun below the navel and 1 cun from the mid-line.	Moxa 5 x.
Sterility (female)	Special point ½ cun outside Ki 13.	Moxa this point with Ki 13 and St 28 bilaterally 7-10 x and needle VC 4.
Malposition of foetus	Bl 67.	Heat for 30 minutes daily until corrected.
Deficient lactation	VC 17, St 18.	Heat 10-20 minutes.
Spermatorrhoea	Special point between Bl 23 and Bl 47.	Moxa this point 7 x, Bl 23 10 x and Bl 47 10 x, bilaterally.
Musculo-skeletal		
Ankle sprained		
—medial aspect	Tip of medial malleolus.	Moxa 3 x or heat 6 minutes.
—lateral aspect	Special point centre of the posterior aspect of the heel at edge of the plantar skin.	Moxa 7 x.
Ganglion	Heat actual swelling.	15-20 minutes. Can use Yuan-Li needle (see p. 63).
Lumbar pain from prolonged standing	Special point lateral to Bl 47 at 4½ cun from the mid-line.	Special technique consisting of 3 large moxa cones blown on to hasten combustion.
Spinal weakness	GV 12.	Meeting point of upper yang.
Spinal deformity	Special points below the inferior edge of 11th rib close to spine level with GV 6.	Moxa 10-20 x, bilaterally.

Condition	*Moxa Treatment*	*Remarks and Rationale*
Chronic spinal disorders	GV 12, Bl 18, Bl 23, Bl 26.	Bl points are Shu points of tissue related organs, e.g., liver (for muscle and connective tissue).
Shoulder joint	Chientungtien, middle of the lateral border of the scapula.	Heat for 10-20 minutes.
—difficulty in elevation	Special point on the acromion between Co 15 and Co 16. Where there is pain on pressure to tip of the acromial process—3 large moxa cones on the tip.	Moxa 7 x and add drainage needle to Co 15 and Co 16. 'Blown' technique to hasten combustion.
—spontaneous dislocation	SI 11, SI 9, TH 13.	Moxa 7 x.
Sciatica	Tip of 5th lumbar vertebra.	Heat for 8-10 minutes and needle special point four fen above Bl 60.
Finger contractures	Points of proximal interphalangeal joints of 1st and 3rd fingers.	Moxa 5 x each.
Rheumatism of fingers	Point of distal interphalangeal joint of affected finger.	
Knee weakness	Apex of patella and St 35. Line across joint just below patella from lateral to medial margins of joint (Hsiyen points).	Heat 3 minutes each. Spreading technique with moxa roll (see p.).
—cold knees	Bl 31.	Also spreading technique.
Hemiplegia	On leg, special point on posterior aspect of lateral malleolus between tip of malleolus and Bl 60. On arm, special point on the ulnar styloid ½ cun above SI 5.	Moxa these points at least 50 x each preferably with a greenstick peck technique. Add 3-5 moxas on Bl 60 and/or SI 6 as called for.

Condition	*Moxa Treatment*	*Remarks and Rationale*
Mental and Neurological		
Spinal cord and brain	Bilateral point at ¾ of the distance from GV 12 to Bl 13.	Moxa 10-30 x GV 12 and 40-70 x each special point.
Convulsions	Centre of plantar crease of hallux. Dorsal foot, immediately proximal to Li 2.	Moxa 5-7 x each, add drainage to Lu 11, Sp 1 and bleed the Bafeng point in the web between the thumb and first finger.
Epilepsy		
—during day	GV 20, VC 15, VC 13, HC 7, Bl 62.	
—at night	Ki 6.	
—general	VC 16.	Moxa 7 x to produce a burn, simultaneously drain SI 5 with a needle bilaterally. (Do not repeat the treatment until the burn has healed.)
Psychosis	Utilizes 6 points very close together. Principal centre is tip of the spinous process of the 2nd dorsal vertebra; immediately above and below it are two other points, whilst there are two further points to the left and right of the inferior point. The apex of the combination is GV 13.	Moxa GV 13 5 x and each of the five special points once for each year of age to a maximum of 40 (see below). 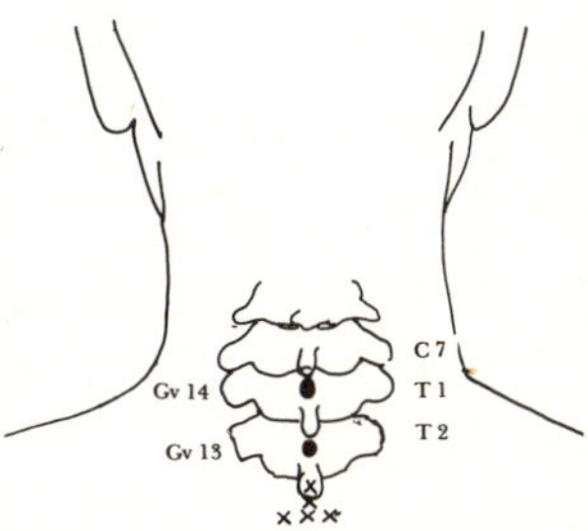
	Special point between Ki 7 and Ki 8.	Moxa 7 x daily for 4 days.
Schizophrenia		
—manic types	GV 20.	
—hallucinations	SI 16.	

Condition	*Moxa Treatment*	*Remarks and Rationale*
Miscellaneous		
Eye conditions	Lateral border of the metacarpo-phalangeal joint of the thumb.	Moxa 3 x.
	Tip of the M-P joint on the thumb.	Moxa 7 x, large cones, 'blown' technique.
Cataract (to augment other treatments)	GV 4.	Not in male under 20.
Epistaxis	GV 23.	
Toothache		
—upper jaw	Point of ulnar styloid just proximal to SI 5.	Use opposite side.
—lower jaw	Point between HC 5 and HC 6.	
Diabetes	Bl 27.	Heavy moxa.
	Tips of the little fingers and toes.	Moxa stick for general heating.
	Cervical vertebrae from atlas to C 7.	
	Special point ½ cun to right of VC 9.	Moxa according to age.
Fainting	GV 20, VC 6.	
Food poisoning	Mark the tip of the second toe with gentian, violet or other transferable stain, flex the toe strongly and, where it touches the metatarsophalangeal area of the foot, moxa according to age.	
Furunculosis	2 unilateral points, utilizing the left hand for a man and the right for a woman: (a) special point on the Ht meridian ¼ cun above Ht 7. (b) Co 4.	Moxa 7 x each.

Condition	*Moxa Treatment*	*Remarks and Rationale*
Goitre — iodine deficiency	—VC 17. —Then VC 22, Bl 7, Lu 2, Co 14, Co 11, Li 4, GB 20, GV 14, St 11, TH 13, Co 3, St 42.	Moxa 7 x. All to be moxa 'd 18 x.
—hyperthyr-oidism	Lu 3.	Moxa 50 x.
Haematemesis	Ki 7, Lu 5, Lu 6, Co 10.	Moxa 3-7 x.
General weakness	Crease formed between the sacrum and the ilium when the patient is standing.	Moxa the lower point of this crease 7-11 x.
—weakness (due to Yang deficiency and Yin excess)	GV 4, Bl 23, Bl 15, VC 4.	
—generally cold and tired	VC 8, VC 4, St 36, Ki 3.	
—to stimulate general Yang energy	GV 14, Co 11, Co 4.	
—lack of energy in the lower part of the body	St 39.	Sea of Blood point.
—to stimulate general energy	St 36.	

APPENDIX 1

FORBIDDEN POINTS AND CONTRA-INDICATIONS TO MOXIBUSTION

Forbidden Points

Lu 3, 8, 10
Co 19, 20
St 7, 8, 9, 17, 32
Sp 1, 7, 19
Ht 6
SI 18
Bl 1, 2, 3, 5, 6, 30, 50, 51, 54, 62
TH 4, 16, 18, 23
GB 5, 15, 22, 33, 42
GV 6, 7, 15, 16, 17, 18, 25
VC 4

The majority of these points are forbidden for cosmetic reasons, i.e., points on the face which might scar, or points in the region of anatomically delicate structures such as the eyes or superficial arteries. Other points are forbidden because of the strong effect they can have on the body's energies. Some, such as TH 4, though forbidden to ordinary moxa, can be particularly effective when used with heated needles, whilst VC 4, though traditionally forbidden, is actually used frequently.

Contra-indications to Moxibustion

1. Forbidden points (see above) with certain exceptions noted in therapeutic repertory.

2. Around the eyes, or on face generally. Anywhere where inadvertant scarring could cause disfigurement.
3. Over superficial blood vessels and varicose veins.
4. Ulcerations or ischaemic areas—anywhere that burning could produce a lesion which would be difficult to heal.
5. Diabetes. Use moxa only with the greatest care since the skin heals with difficulty in this condition and there is often a degree of loss of sensory appreciation.
6. Hypoaesthesia. For example following cerebrovascular accident and neurological damage.
7. Oedematous tissues. Overtly oedematous areas must be avoided because of the poor healing capacity and loss of sensation.
8. Hypertension. Particular caution in the use of points which move Yang energy upwards, e.g., GV 14.
9. Very young children. Childrens skin is extremely tender and they may not know when it is too hot.
10. The very old. Skin lacks resilience and sensory appreciation may be diminished.

APPENDIX 2

JAPANESE MOXIBUSTION

Moxibustion is used very extensively in Japan and the basic applications are the same as those which apply in China, the main difference being that, where moxa cones are used, the Japanese favour smaller cones, usually rice size. Indirect moxibustion is also applied using large cones on top of a 7mm (¼ in) thick slice of garlic, or on a disc (25mm × 7mm, 1 in × ¼ in) made from a mixture of one part grated garlic to 6 parts miso (bean mush). The cones are burnt until the patient feels the heat.

A slight variation of moxa roll technique, known as *Oshi Gyu* is used. The appropriate points are covered with eight-ply bleached linen, with a sheet of paper on top and the tip of the roll is applied until the patient feels the heat.

The following repertory of treatment formulas is drawn from various Japanese sources.[1 2 3] They generally recommend rice-grain-sized moxa pinches, but the treatment can be effectively carried out using greenstick tapers or moxa rolls.

REPERTORY OF JAPANESE MOXIBUSTION TECHNIQUES

Condition	*Moxa points*	*Remarks*
Bladder		
—pollakiuria, pain along urinary tract, pain on micturition, tenesmus.	VC 3, VC 9, Ki 12, GV 2, GV 3, Bl 32, Bl 33, Sp 10, Li 8, Sp 6, Ki 6	5 x ½ rice-grain-sized cones at each point, or use greenstick taper.
—symptoms acute and severe	VC 3, VC 9, Ki 2, GV 2, GV 3, Bl 32, Bl 33	50-100 x ½ rice-grain-sized cones at each point.
Lumbago and coldness of back and lower legs	Add Bl 23, Bl 47, Ki 2	
Severe coldness of feet and lower extremities	Add Ki 2, GV 33, St 36, GB 34, GB 41, GB 43	GB 33 also used for coldness of entire body.
Boils		
—general, any location	Co 4, Co 10, Co 11 Si 6	Moxa 50-100 x (rice-sized cones). When affected area lies on median line treat bilaterally; otherwise affected side. Can add Co 15.
—upper part of body affected	Add Si 10, Si 11	10 x ½ rice-sized cones.
—lower body or lower extremities	Add Bl 25, Onodera's point.	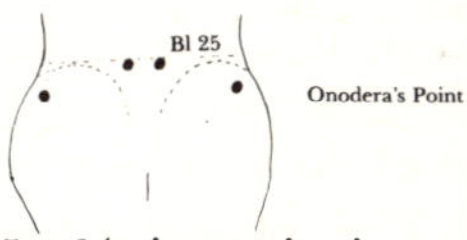
—to balance general bodily functions	GV 12, St 36	5 x ½ rice-grain-size cones.
Brachial paralysis	SI 13, Co 15, Co 11, Co 4. Can add GB 20, SI 10, Co 13, TH 9	Moxa 3-5 x each.
Cervico-brachial syndrome	Si 13, Si 10, Bl 38, TH 13, Co 11, special points Hsiafutu, Chienchien.	Moxa 5 x each.
	or	
	Si 13, Bl 10, Co 11, Hsiafutu, Chienchien.	Heated needle.

Condition	*Moxa Treatment*	*Remarks and Rationale*
Epilepsy	Bl 10, GV 11, Bl 13, GV 21, GB 34	Moxa 5 x. Treat daily for 20 days, rest 14 days and then start a second course.
Facial paralysis	TH 22, GB 20, TH 17, GV 11, Co 11, Bl 13, and Bl 21 *or* Moxa on garlic to St 3, 4, 6, and 7, SI 18, TH 22, Tai Yang.	Moxa 5 x. Treat bilaterally.
Headache	GV 19, GV 11, GB 20, Bl 18, Bl 23, GB 34, Bl 60	
—severe pain	Bl 10, GV 12	Moxa 10-15 x.
—chronic headaches	Bl 10	Moxa regularly for 3-6 months.
Hemiplegia	Bl 18, GB 20, Co 15, Co 11, TH 8, special lateral gluteal point, GB 31, Bl 51, St 36, Bl 56, GB 39	Moxa 5-7 x. Best results if treatment started within 10 days of attack —after 6 months results very poor.
High Blood Pressure		
—essential hypertension	GV 4, VC 9, Sp 8, GV 20, GV 12, TH 15, Bl 32	Very small moxa cones. In serious cases omit Bl 32 and substitute GV 9.
—for insomnia, headache, and heavy headedness	Add GB 20, Ht 7	Avoid treating too many points at one session.
—for tinnitus, dizziness and unsteadiness	Add Ki 5, or Ki 2, Ht 3	
—for palpitations dyspnoea or arrhythmia	Add Ht 7, and HC 4	
—for aphasia add	GV 15	
—arteriosclerosis	As for essential hypertension.	
—coronary sclerosis	Add left Si 12, left Bl 15, left Ht 7 and Ht 3	
—cerebral sclerosis	Add Bl 7, bilaterally.	

Condition	*Moxa Treatment*	*Remarks and Rationale*
—renal sclerosis —intermittent claudication —malignant hypertension	Add Ki 1. Add GB 34, St 36, GB 41, Li 3. VC 9, GV 9, GV 12, GV 20, TH 15.	Confine treatment to these points although others may be indicated.
Hypotension	VC 12, St 21, Co 11, St 36, GV 12, TH 15, Bl 10, Bl 17, Bl 20, Bl 23.	5 very small moxa cones (Sesame seed size) to each point.
Insomnia	GB 2, GB 17, Bl 14, Bl 18, GB 34, VC 12, VC 4	Moxa 5-7 x daily.
Intercostal neuralgia	Bl 14 (bilaterally), Bl 15, Bl 39, GB 22, Ki 23, VC 12.	Moxa 5 x each, if tender up to 15 x.
Leucoderma —pea-sized or smaller area —large areas	GV 12, Bl 20, Bl 32, TH 15, Co 15, Co 10, Co 11, and at centre of affected area. Plum Blossom Needling at 5 points one cm away from the area, plus moxa as above.	5 x ½ rice-grain cones. Treat daily for 5 days, rest for 10, then repeat. Best used in conjunction with Plum Blossom Needle. Dietary and constitutional treatment essential.
Lumbago —upper lumbar —middle lumbar —lumbo-sacral area	GB 31, Bl 56, Bl 60 *plus* Bl 23, Bl 47. Bl 23, Bl 24, Bl 25 Yangkuan (medial to Bl 25), Bl 31.	Moxa 5 x each.
Neurosis	GB 20, GV 11, Bl 14, Bl 18, Bl 23, VC 12, GB 34, Sp 6.	Moxa 3-5 x. Long term treatment.

Condition	*Moxa Treatment*	*Remarks and Rationale*
Nephritis and nephrosis	VC 3, VC 9, Li 8, Co 11, GV 12, Bl 32.	Very fine small cones.
—with high blood pressure (over 160/95), headache and heavy headedness	Add GV 20, GB 20	
—with stiff shoulders	Add TH 15	
—with loss of appetite or other Gastro-intestinal disturbance	Add VC 12, Bl 17, Bl 20	
Pyelitis		
—general treatment	VC 3, VC 9, Bl 20, Bl 23, Bl 47, Ki 1	5 sesame-seed-sized cones at each point.
—with lumbago or backache	Add GV 12, Bl 17, Bl 18	
—with vomiting or loss of appetite	Add VC 12, Bl 45	
—with headache or insomnia	Add GB 20, GV 20	
— with fever or general fatigue	Add SI 3	
Ringworm		
—trichophytia, capilitti and trichophytia facialis	Co 11, Co 15.	5 sesame-seed-sized cones, once daily for a month.
—T. pompholyciformis on fingers	Co 10, Co 11, Co 15, HC 4, HC 7, TH 4, GV 12.	5 x ½ rice-sized cones burnt daily on each point.
—when toes are affected	GB 40, Ki 6, Sp 4.	
—larger areas	Points on and around the area selected to enclose it.	This treatment may also be used for eczema.
Sexual weakness (male)	VC 2, VC 3, VC 4, Ki 12, GV 3, Bl 23, Bl 32, Bl 33.	5 x ½ rice-sized cones daily at each point.
Tachycardia	VC 17, Ht 3, Ht 7, GB 34, GV 9, GV 12, TH 15, SI 11, Sp 8, HC 4.	5 sesame seed-sized cones at each point.

Condition	*Moxa Treatment*	*Remarks and Rationale*
—with cardiac dilatation or hypertrophy —with high blood pressure or arteriosclerosis —with hyperactivity of thyroid gland	Add Ki 27 and HC 1. Omit Sp 8. Add Ki 27, and Ki 6.	
Urticaria	Co 10, Co 11, Co 15, TH 15, GV 9, GV 12.	5 x ½ rice-sized cones.
Verrucae (warts)	20-30 rice-sized cones burnt directly on the wart once daily for 3 days. If one course of treatment does not completely remove the wart repeat 2-3 times.	
V. plana juveniles	Locate parent growth, i.e., largest wart, and administer 20-30 rice-sized cones directly on this wart. After this growth is removed others will also disappear.	

REFERENCES

[1]Kinoshita, H., 'Neuropathy', Vol. 1, *Modern Acupuncture and Moxibustion Series* (Ido-No-Nippon-Sha, Yokosuka, 1973).

[2]Mori, H., 'Diseases of the Locomotor Apparatus', Vol. 3 of *Modern Acupuncture and Moxibustion Series* (Ido-No-Nippon-Sha, Yokosuka, 1974).

[3]Kurashima, S., 'Circulatory, Renal, and Skin Diseases', Vol. 4 of *Modern Acupuncture and Moxibustion Series* (Ido-No-Nippon-Sha, Yokosuka, 1976).

APPENDIX 3

AKABANE TEST

This test, named after its Japanese originator, Dr Kobei Akabane, is a method of determining the energetic equilibrium of the individual meridians by comparing their response to the application of heat at their Tsing points.

The heat is applied by a glowing greenstick taper (hence often known as an Akabane stick) with a technique rather similar to the 'pecking' method, except that the taper is moved in a regular sweep from the centre of the nail out over the Tsing point and back again, each complete return sweep being counted as one application.

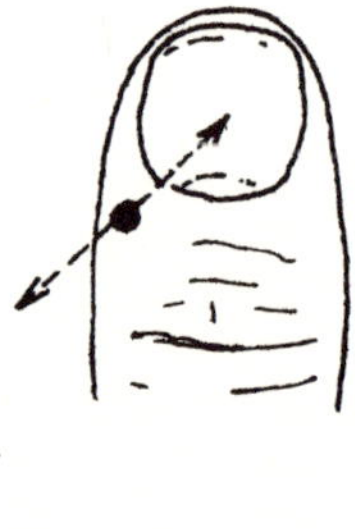

The patient is requested to stand the heat until it suddenly starts to prick at the limit of tolerance, and the number of applications required to reach this limit is counted and recorded. It is best to perform every test in the same manner, starting with the left hand and continuing with the same meridian on the right hand, then the next meridian on the left hand and so on, in the order of the 24 hour cycle, and to write the results down with the left hand on top, as in: Lu 7/8; Co 9/11; St 14/11; Sp 12/10.

It will be realized that the point having the highest reading (i.e., requiring the greatest number of applications to reach tolerance limit) will be the point most *deficient* in energy, and vice versa.

In practical usage, one can safely assume that the number of applications required in the average patient will be about ten. A highly sensitive patient will give a reading of between three and six, whilst a hypoactive patient will show readings of between twelve and eighteen. A quick glance at the overall picture will thus determine the patient's degree of hyper- or hypo-activity, and the state of the individual meridians will be obvious on slightly closer inspection.

The greatest usefulness of this test is that (unlike the pulses) it can show up imbalances between the left and right side meridians.

It will also be realized that the manner of application is really rather imprecise — the operator must endeavour to keep the taper at exactly the same distance above each point — usually about ⅛ in, and to keep each sweep as equal as possible, whilst the patient must be instructed to say 'now' when the same degree of heat is reached on each of the points. These variations are compensated for by considering that a definite imbalance exists only when the reading for one side of a meridian is twice or more that for the opposite side, i.e., 3/6; 14/6, 9/19, or similar, and quite definite diagnoses can be made from this method. A typical reading might be

Ht 4/5; Si 5/6; GB 3/5; Li 8/7; HC 7/6; TH 4/6

in a case of left-sided migraine. Here, the patient is generally hyperactive, but there is a particular sensitivity on the left GB meridian, although there is no complete imbalance between the left and right GB.

Interesting questions, however, spring to mind when it is found that the Akabane test is at complete variance with the pulse picture! This has frequently been found to be the case, and has led one of us (R.L.) to formulate the hypothesis that the pulse gives the state of the organ and Akabane the state of the meridians. But this is a purely personal opinion and there is yet much work to be done on this aspect.

Attempts to render the test more precise have resulted in the development of a special spring device (see drawing) which is supposed to keep the tip of the taper at a controlled distance above the skin. However, frequent adjustment is required to overcome the build-up of ash and concomitant shortening of the stick through burning, and this in itself practically neutralizes the benefits the device is assumed to produce. Various means of producing electrical heating at controlled temperatures are also available.

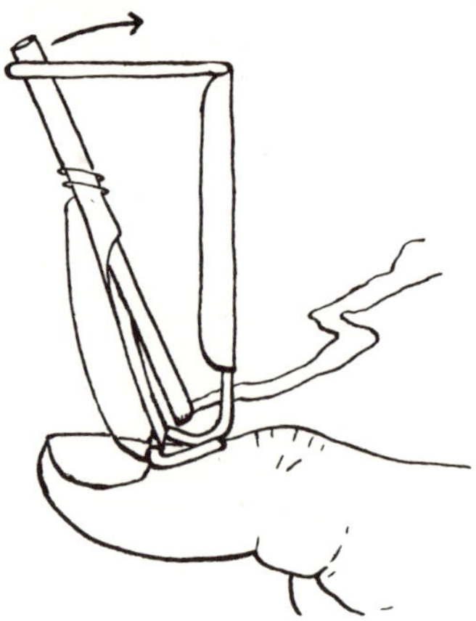

Akabane testing device

Some allowance has to be made for the presence of acute pain in a limb, which could modify the response towards Yang or excess in the meridians of that limb whilst, in the case of the Bladder meridian, the presence of a Durlacher's corn with resultant hard skin over Bl 67 could make a definitive result for that particular meridian almost impossible to obtain.

It must be noted that for the purpose of the test Ki 1 is placed at the medial corner of the nail of the fifth toe (nearest the fourth toe).

APPENDIX 4

CUPPING

This form of treatment, known as 'Bahuoguan' or 'Xifong', has long been associated with traditional methods of acupuncture. As it involves the use of heat it is generally considered in relation to moxibustion although, by contrast, its principle is one of draining areas of congestion, and excess, or perverse energy. In Europe, where it is known as 'Humoral Therapy', cupping has also been widely practised using both wet and dry techniques.

Vessels made of bamboo, earthenware, copper, iron, or glass are used. To suck out the air paper or cotton is ignited and placed inside the cup, then removed with forceps. The cup is immediately placed over the point with the lips downwards and the vacuum created exerts a suction on the flesh around the point.

Dry cupping is the use of suction only for 10-15 minutes. In wet cupping the points are made to bleed with a Plum Blossom (Seven Star) needle, or a prismatic needle, and the cup is then applied to draw the blood by its suction.

The cup is removed by pressing the surrounding flesh to let air in. Cupping techniques are most suitable for stout, full-blooded patients. They are generally applied to hairless areas, back, shoulders, abdomen, or thighs, and can be used after acupuncture. The following conditions respond well to cupping techniques applied to the indicated points.

Lumbago	—	Bl 23, Bl 47
Abdominal pain	—	VC 12, St 25
Asthma	—	Bl 13
Scapulo-humeral neuralgia	—	Local points
Headaches	—	Taiyang
Rheumatism	—	Local points

APPENDIX 5

GROW YOUR OWN MOXA

by Royston Low

The plant Mugwort (*Artemisia vulgaris*) is readily grown in England — in fact, it can be found as a perennial weed growing on waste-land and in hedgerows over the greater part of the country. It usually grows to a height of from three to five feet and is most often found in large clumps.

Traditionally it is the leaves alone which are used, but I have found that the minute 'flowers' can also be added to good effect — they aid the felting and also add to the amount of punk available. To this end I harvest the crop when the seeds are just about forming, usually from the middle of July to the middle of August.

The stems are cut through at the level of the lowest leaves and are then placed in drying racks in an airy place for about two years. They should not be piled too heavily on top of each other as the idea is to let air get to the leaves so that they can dry out naturally — too large a pile and there is danger of mould forming, which would ruin the crop completely. The layers are turned over every couple of months or so to assist the general drying. At the end of the two years the plants are ready for use, and the dried leaves and 'flowers' are just shredded off the stems into a large cardboard box for transfer to the stock-room (see illustration 1).

To manufacture the actual punk, a handful of leaves is crumpled up and placed in an electric coffee-grinder (being careful to remove any pieces of woody mid-rib and small twigs) (see illustration 2) and ground for about twenty seconds, this being about the optimum time (see illustration 3). The contents are then tipped out into a fine flour-sieve and the dust sifted out (see illustrations 4 and 5). The resultant punk is ready for use (see illustration 6).

Experience has proved that one cannot prepare a very large amount at one time, as the electric grinder may over-heat. I tend to prepare two lots of punk, then put them both back into the grinder together with a small amount of the Chinese punk to alter the texture slightly, and then grind for a further ten seconds. I find this gives me enough punk to last for perhaps ten or twelve treatments, and takes only a maximum of five minutes overall to prepare.

The advantage of this method is that, apart from having a constant supply of punk available, the finished product is superior to imported punk and one can, with experiment, determine the grade of fineness and felting which best suits one's own needs.

The disadvantages are the finding of suitable space for the drying racks (I suspend mine inside the roof of my garage!) and the fact that one has to think two years ahead in terms of availability. There is no trouble at all in growing it—a piece of land ten feet by five will easily grow enough for each year's crop, and if this should run low, a visit to some local waste-land will frequently yield further supplies. It can easily be grown from seed, although this will need to be obtained from specialist herb-growers, but the easiest way to start off is to acquire a few roots. They will soon establish themselves, flourish and spread.

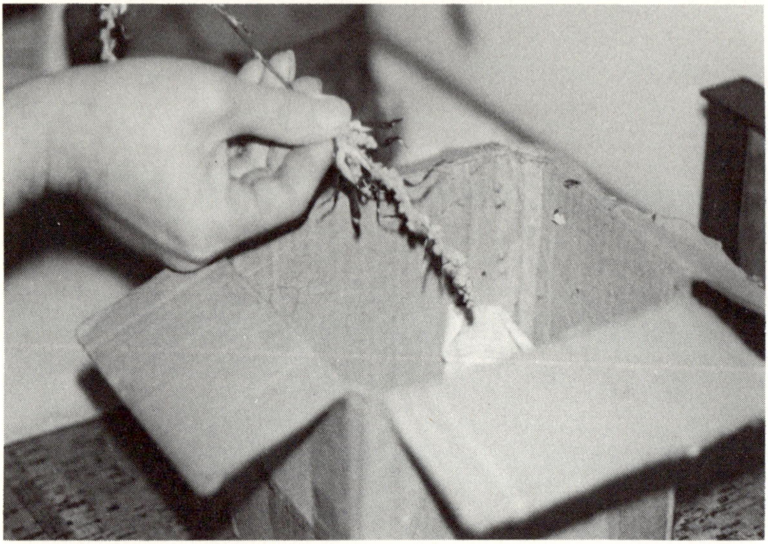

1. *Artemisia vulgaris* plant, which has been dried for a minimum of two years, is stripped of the leaves and flower heads, which are collected in a cardboard box.

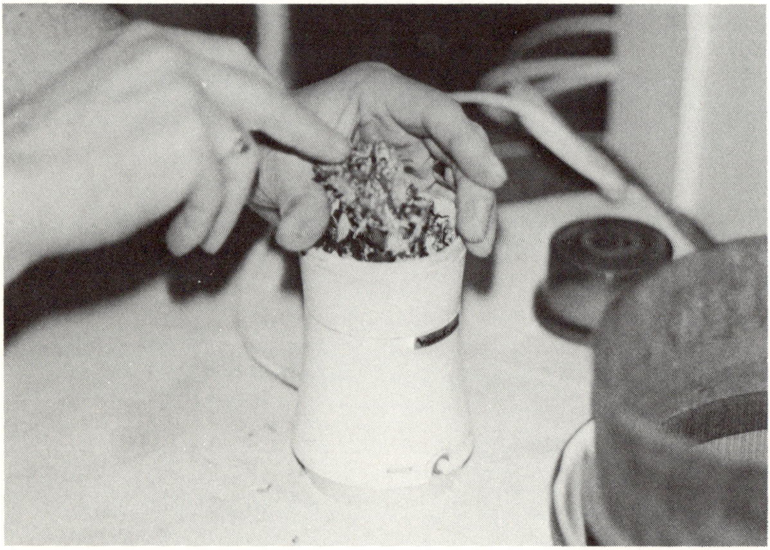

2. The dried leaves and flowers are crumpled up and placed in a coffee grinder. Woody midribs and twigs must be removed.

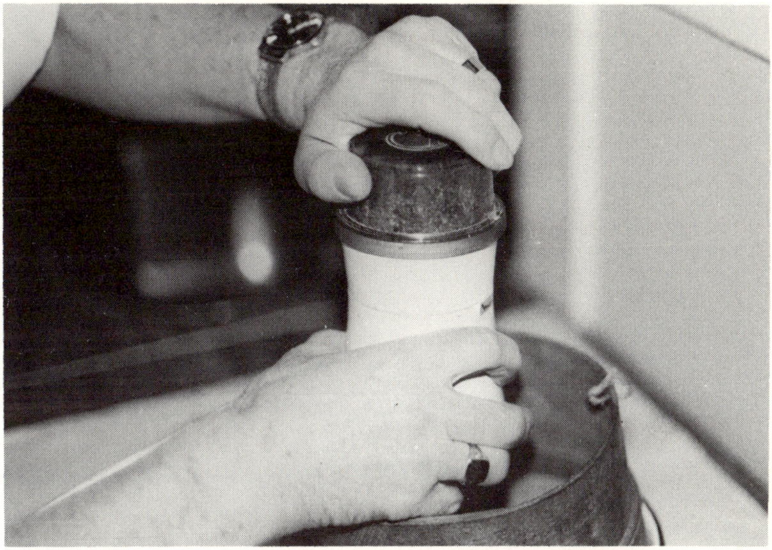

3. The dried herb is ground for approximately 20 seconds.

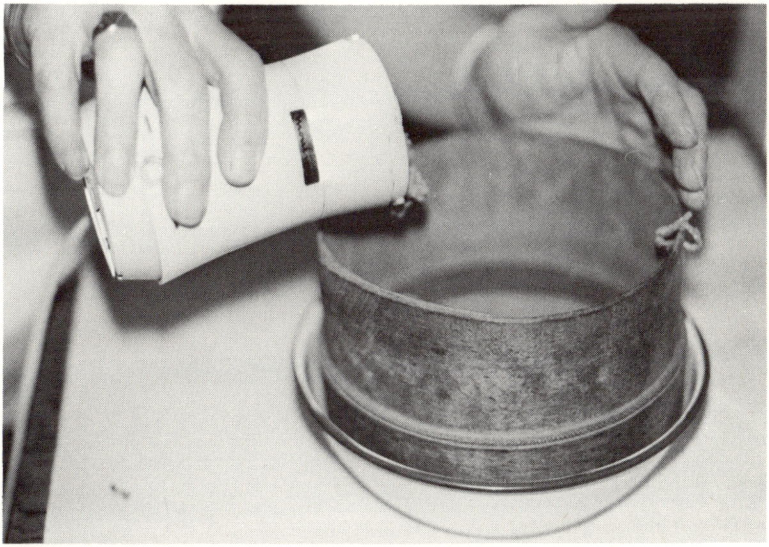

4. The resultant moxa wool is placed in a sieve . . .

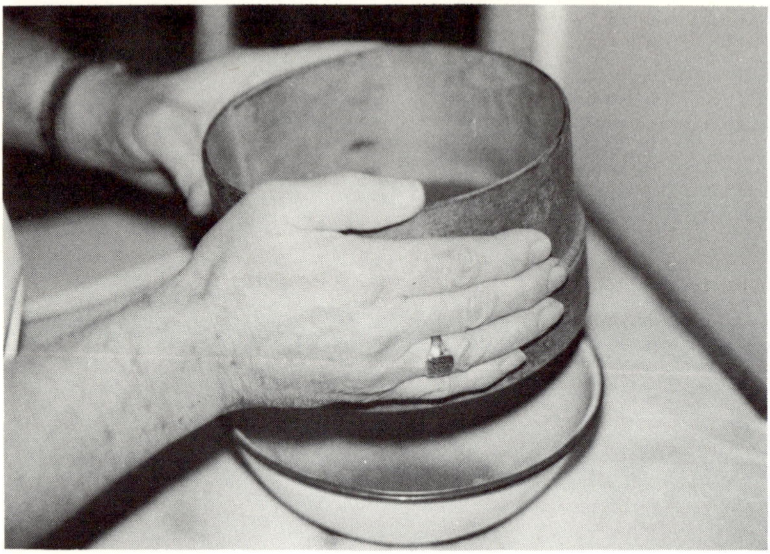

5. . . . and shaken to remove dust and fine particles.

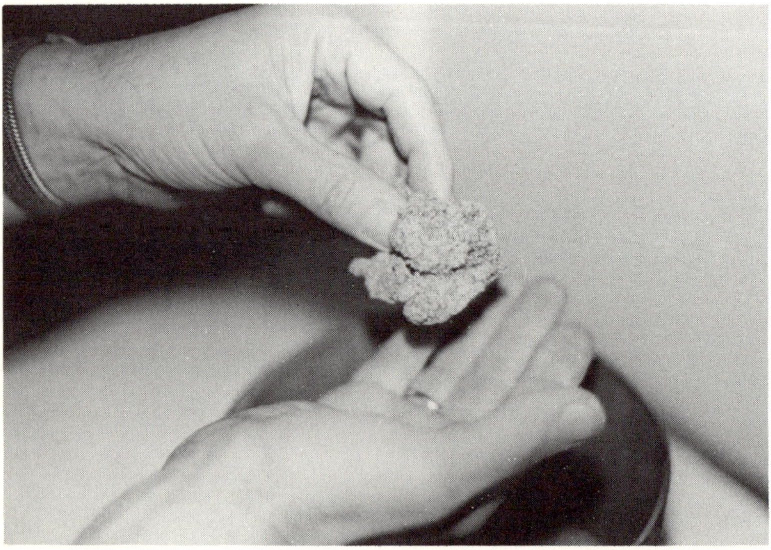

6. The remaining moxa wool, or punk, has a fine spongy consistency ready for use.

GLOSSARY

Acupuncture and moxibustion have come to the west from many Eastern sources with the result that the terminology in use can be a confusing mixture of different languages. Furthermore the current modernization of the various Chinese dialects towards the standard Pinyin has left even comparatively up-to-date texts with an older terminology still in use.

We have tried, as far as possible in this book, to be consistent in our terminology and keep to Pinyin or Mandarin Chinese, except where such spelling would represent a break with established usage. Experienced acupuncturists will forgive the occasional lapse of authors long-accustomed to Wade-Giles, or other romanization, and recognize the appropriate terms without difficulty. Where passages from other publications have been quoted the original spelling used by the author has been retained and may differ from that used in the main body of our text.

Meridians

The standard Western terminology, being the least confusing, and the universally accepted system of numbering each channel from point one upwards, are adopted throughout this text. The following abbreviations have been used:

Lu — Lung
Co — Colon or large intestine
St — Stomach
Sp — Spleen/pancreas
Ht — Heart

SI — Small intestine
Bl — Bladder
Ki — Kidney
HC — Heart constrictor or circulation/sex
TH — Three heater or triple warmer
GB — Gall bladder
Li — Liver
GV — Governor vessel
VC — Vessel of conception

Command Points

Tsing
Yong
Yu
Yuen
Ching
Ho

Irregular Vessels (Eight extra meridians)

Du mo — Governor vessel
Ren mo — Conception vessel
Yang keo mo — Yang vessel of ankle
Yin keo mo — Yin vessel of ankle
Dai mo — Vessel of the waist
Chong mo — Vessel of the groin
Yin wei mo — Vessel reuniting the yin
Yang wei mo — Vessel reuniting the yang

The Six Chaos

Tai yang — SI, Bl
Chao yang — TH, GB
Yang ming — Co, St
Tai yin — Lu, Sp
Tsieu yin — HC, Li
Chao yin — Ht, Ki

Perverse Energies

Wind — Fong
Cold — Han
Heat — Shu
Humidity — Shih

Dryness	— Zao
Fire	— Huo

Units of Measurement

1 cun	= 10 fen

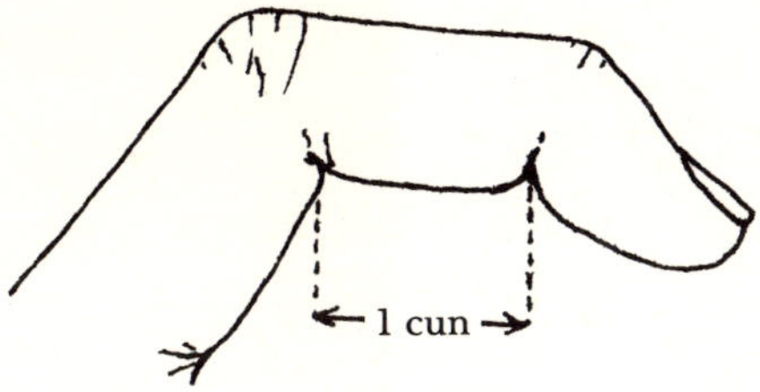

Index finger of patient

INDEX